more advance praise for
How to Be Sick

"This is a book for all of us."
—SYLVIA BOORSTEIN,
author of *Happiness Is an Inside Job*

"An immensely wise book. Health psychology has been poisoned by the view that the best way to approach illness is through a muscular, militant resistance. Toni Bernhard reveals how letting go, surrendering, and putting the ego aside yield insights and fulfillment even in the presence of illness. A major contribution."
—LARRY DOSSEY, MD,
author of *The Power of Premonitions* and *Healing Words*

"Everyone should read this book—anyone who is sick, anyone who loves someone who is sick, and anyone who has ever experienced things being other than they'd hoped they would be. Toni Bernhard open-heartedly shares the deep pain and equally deep joy of her experience in a way that allows us to validate the pain of our own circumstances, and still find joy and contentment within any context. She offers simple, deeply wise practices that reduce the suffering associated with grasping for things to be other than they are by allowing us to accept and enjoy things exactly as they are, including our own desire for something else. Her willingness to step fully into her life after it's been dramatically narrowed by illness, and to share this process with us, inspires us each to live our own lives more fully, accepting the challenges that arise, and finding the joys inherent in each moment. Toni's writing feels like a good friend, helping us cultivate compassion for ourselves and those around us, as we make our way through whatever life presents to us. Her honesty in sharing her struggles and setbacks helps us be kinder to ourselves as we experience our own. I plan to buy a copy for everyone I love."
—LIZABETH ROEMER, PHD,
co-author of *The Mindful Way through Anxiety*

continued...

"This warm and engaging book can help with
even the most difficult situation."
—THOMAS BIEN, PhD, author of *Mindful Therapy*

"*How To Be Sick* is a good friend to keep close by so that illness
doesn't become the enemy."
—ED & DEB SHAPIRO, authors of *Be the Change*

"Don't pass up this book—and don't be misled by the title. This
book isn't about being sick as much as it as about living right
now. This practical yet exceedingly graceful book is a love story—
about life, the endurance of the human spirit, and the power of a
sustaining relationship."
—ALIDA BRILL, author of *Dancing at the River's Edge*

"Living a life of peace and contentment is not difficult when life is
cooperating—but what happens when the reality of our lives is
suddenly turned upside down and shaken by hardship or
affliction? This book is an inspiring and instructive guide for
coping with a chronic condition or life-threatening illness but it is
much more than that. Each chapter is about unpacking the highest
truth in the lowest places of our lives.
The book is called *How To Be Sick* but it's really about how to live."
—JIM PALMER, author of *Divine Nobodies*

"An intimate, gripping, profound, and eminently useful book about
being joyfully and wisely alive no matter what happens to you."
—RICK HANSON, PHD, author of *Buddha's Brain*

"Who would have thought that there is a 'how to' for being sick?
But now there is! Deeply moving and impressive. I highly
recommend her book as a must-read for anyone who is ill or
caring for someone ill. Her gifts will transform you."
—LEWIS RICHMOND, author of *Healing Lazarus*

continued...

How to Be Sick

A Buddhist-Inspired Guide
for the Chronically Ill
and their Caregivers

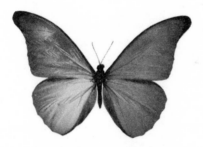

Toni Bernhard

WISDOM PUBLICATIONS • BOSTON

Wisdom Publications
199 Elm Street
Somerville MA 02144 USA
www.wisdompubs.org

Library of Congress Cataloging-in-Publication Data
Bernhard, Toni.
  How to be sick : a Buddhist-inspired guide for the chronically ill and their caregivers /
Toni Bernhard.
     p. cm.
  Includes bibliographical references and index.
  ISBN 0-86171-626-4 (pbk. : alk. paper)
  1. Religious life—Buddhism. 2. Chronically ill—Religious life. 3. Caregivers—Religious
life. 4. Chronic diseases—Religious aspects—Buddhism. I. Title.
  BQ5400.B46 2010
  294.3'4442—dc22

                              2010025648

18 17 16 15 14   8 7 6 5 4

ISBN 978-0-86171-626-5   eBook ISBN 978-0-86171-926-6

Cover design by Phil Pascuzzo. Interior design by Gopa&Ted2, Inc. Set in Sabon LT Std
11/16.

Wisdom Publications' books are printed on acid-free paper and meet the guidelines for
permanence and durability of the Production Guidelines for Book Longevity of the
Council on Library Resources.

This book was produced with environmental mindfulness. We have elected to print this
title on 30% PCW recycled paper. As a result, we have saved the following resources:
15 trees, 6 million BTUs of energy, 1,323 lbs. of greenhouse gases, 7,176 gallons of
water, and 480 lbs. of solid waste. For more information, please visit our website,
www.wisdompubs.org.

Printed in the United States of America.

MIX
Paper from
responsible sources
FSC
www.fsc.org   FSC® C011935

For more information: visit www.fscus.org.

For Tony

In sickness and in health,
to love and to cherish,
till death do us part.

Table of Contents

Turnarounds and Transformations

From Isolation to Solitude

Foreword

"YOU ARE GOING TO BE OKAY!" Words of reassurance are the first therapy offered to people who awaken after a surgery, or are revived after an accident, or just before the disclosure of a fearful diagnosis. "You are going to be okay" often goes along with the summary of what now needs to happen to make things better. "You'll need to stay a few more days in the hospital and then you can go home and finish recuperating there." Or, "We're on the way to the hospital and the doctors there are ready for you." Or, "We'll do chemo and then radiation and it might be a hard year but the chances are good that you'll be your old self again afterward." "You are going to be okay," in these circumstances, means "Things are uncomfortable now, but you will get well. You will be better." But it doesn't always happen that way.

This is a book for people who will not be their old self again and for all those for whom, at least now, getting better *isn't* possible. This is a book that most reassuringly says even to those people, "You, too, are going to be okay—even if you never recover your health!"

Toni Bernhard is the perfect person to write this book. In the middle of a vibrant, complex, gratifying family and professional life—literally from one day to the next—she took ill with a hard-to-diagnose and basically incurable, painfully fatiguing illness that waxes and wanes in its intensity, that sometimes seems to respond to a new treatment and then doesn't after all, that doesn't get worse but also never gets better. Nine years after the onset of her illness, she is still sick. She knows the cycle of hoping and feeling disappointed from the inside out as well as the cycles of deciding to give up hope in order to avoid the pain of disappointment and the sadness, and then the relief, of surrender.

Decades ago, a friend of mine, a man with a family and friends and flourishing career, said of his unexpected, debilitating illness, "This isn't what I wanted—but it's what I got." He said it matter-of-factly, without bitterness, as if he understood that it was the only reasonable response. I knew that he was telling me something important. It is a fundamental human truth, transcending cultures and traditions, that the wisest response to situations that are beyond our control, circumstances that we cannot change, is noncontention. In this book, Toni shows how her longtime study and meditation practice in the Buddhist tradition help her accommodate her situation with gentle acceptance and compassion. The techniques that Toni presents for working with one's mind in the distressed states it finds itself when facing an uncomfortable and unchangeable truth are basic Buddhist insights and meditation practices, but they are nonparochial. They will work for anyone.

This book is written for people who are ill and aren't going to get better, and also for their caregivers, people who love them and suffer along with them in wishing that things were different. It speaks most specifically about physical illness. In the largest sense, though, I feel that this book is for all of us. Sooner or later, we all are all going to not "get better." Speaking as an older person who has had the good fortune of health, I know that the core challenge in my life, and, I believe, in all of our lives, from beginning to end, is accommodating to realities that we wish were other, and doing it with grace.

Toni has given us a gift by sharing her life and her wisdom and I am grateful for it.

—Sylvia Boorstein

Preface

One, seven, three, five—
Nothing to rely on in this or any world;
Nighttime falls and the water is flooded with moonlight.
Here in the Dragon's jaws:
Many exquisite jewels.

—SETCHO JUKEN

IN MAY OF 2001, I GOT SICK AND NEVER RECOVERED.
The summer of 2008 marked my seventh year of living with chronic illness. One night that summer, at about 10:00 P.M., my husband came into our bedroom and joined me on the bed that has become my home. My husband's parents named him Tony; my parents named me Toni. We met when we were dating each other's roommates in college. On the morning of November 22, 1963, he knocked on my apartment door with the news that President Kennedy had been shot. Tony and I have been inseparable ever since. By this time of night, I'm in what we call "stun-gun" state—as if I'd been hit with a Taser—meaning it's often hard for me to move my body and do anything other than stare blankly into space.

I greeted him with, "I wish I weren't sick."

Tony replied, "I wish you weren't sick."

There was a slight pause, then we both started laughing.

"Okay. That got said."

It was a breakthrough moment for the two of us.

We'd had this exchange dozens of times since the summer of 2001, but it took seven long years for the exchange to bring us to laughter instead of to sorrow and, often, to tears. This book tells the story of how Tony and I moved from tears to laughter. Not always laughter, of course, but laughter enough.

I've written *How to Be Sick* to help and inspire the chronically ill and their caregivers as they meet the challenges posed by any chronic illness or condition, including:

- coping with symptoms that just won't go away
- coming to terms with a more isolated life
- weathering fear about the future
- facing the misunderstanding of others
- dealing with the health care system; and
- for spouses, partners, or other caregivers, adapting to so many unexpected and sometimes sudden life changes.

In chapters 1 and 2, I talk about how I got sick and, to Tony's and my own bewilderment, stayed sick. Starting in chapter 3, I describe how, drawing on the teachings of the Buddha (often called the Dharma), I learned the spiritual practice of "how to be sick," meaning how to live a life of equanimity and joy despite my physical and energetic limitations. I offer simple practices, ranging from those that are traditionally Buddhist to others I devised after becoming chronically ill. I also include a chapter on Byron Katie's work, which I have found particularly helpful.

You need not be a Buddhist to benefit from the practices in this book. If a suggested practice resonates with you, truly "practice" it. Work with it over and over until it enters your heart, mind, and body and becomes a natural response to the difficulties you face as the result of being chronically ill or being the caregiver of a chronically ill person.

At the end of the book, I've provided a quick reference guide that matches specific challenges faced by the chronically ill and their caregivers to practices described in the book.

I put this book together slowly and with great difficulty. I wrote it lying on my bed, laptop on my stomach, notes strewn about on the blanket, printer within arm's reach. Some days I would get so involved in a chapter that I'd work too long. The result would be an exacerbation of my symptoms that would leave me unable to write at all for several days or even for weeks.

There were also periods when I was simply too sick to even think of putting a book together. Then the project would be left untouched for months on end. Being so physically sick would sometimes have such a strong effect on my mental state that, during the darkest moments, I considered tossing out all the work I'd done, despairing of ever being able to complete it.

But mental states come and go—and in the end, I pressed on, determined to finish the book in the hope it would help others. The Buddha's teachings have inspired and comforted me during this illness. The Buddha and the schools that his teachings gave rise to offer many simple and helpful practices that guide both the healthy and the sick through life's ups and downs.

The inspiration to write this book came from a person I knew for such a short time and in such limited circumstances that I don't even know how to spell her name. In 1999, I was on a ten-day silent meditation retreat at Spirit Rock Meditation Center. As always on retreat, each of us had what's called "work meditation," meaning we are responsible for performing a task each day to help the retreat run smoothly. Some people cut vegetables, some wash dishes, others clean the bathrooms. As much as possible, we maintain silence even if we work alongside others.

My work meditation was to clear the trays from the serving tables in the dining hall after lunch and put the leftovers in containers. I shared this job with a woman who introduced herself as Marianne and was about my age. She looked a bit frail to me, but we shared the work equally, only speaking in a whisper now and then: "Is this container big enough to hold the extra salad?" In the meditation hall, I noticed that she seemed to be with a young man who might be her son. I remember thinking how nice it was that they were here together. She had a kind face and a gentle smile and I looked forward to seeing her every day after lunch.

In addition to working in the dining hall, we followed a path to a small building where the teachers ate and then we brought their serving trays back to the kitchen. On the seventh day of the retreat, to my surprise, another woman accompanied my partner. The three of us cleared the serving tables in the dining hall and then the new woman followed me outside as I began to walk down to the teachers' dining room. She asked, "Do you know about Marianne?"

When I shook my head, she told me, "She's very sick. She only has a couple of weeks to live." Then, she turned around and went back into the dining hall.

I continued to the teachers' dining room, shaken by this unexpected discovery. The room was empty, but the *San Francisco Chronicle* was on the table where the teachers ate. (I was on retreat, but the teachers weren't and so newspapers were always scattered about on the table. I'd learned to avert my eyes.) But the *Chronicle* that day had a headline in letters too bold to ignore:

Having no idea what the backstory was, I quickly left the room in shock, my heart pounding, my mind spinning. There, on the path, was one of the teachers. In my distress, I broke the silence. She briefly told me what had happened to JFK Jr. (and also commented that they shouldn't leave newspapers lying around). I asked her if she knew about Marianne. She told me Marianne was here with her son. Then she told me something she probably shouldn't have (which is why I'm not using her name). She said that on the information sheet we fill out when we get to the retreat, under the question that asks if there's anything the teachers should know about us, Marianne had written, "I have just two weeks to live but it won't affect my practice."

The next day Marianne's spot and her son's spot in the meditation hall were empty.

In memory of Marianne, I vow to do my best not to let my illness affect my practice. I also vow to let my practice continue to teach me how to be sick—and to enable me to help others who are chronically ill.

How Everything Changed

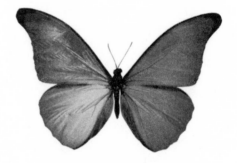

I

Getting Sick: A Romantic Trip to Paris

Paris ain't much of a town.

—BABE RUTH

AT THE END OF AUGUST 2001, I was to begin my twentieth year as a law professor at the University of California at Davis. To celebrate and to treat ourselves, Tony and I decided to go on a special vacation. Surfing the Internet, I found a studio apartment to rent in Paris at a reasonable rate. We were not world travelers: a trip to Paris was a big deal for us. For three weeks, we'd immerse ourselves in the life and culture of the City of Lights. We were going to have a great time.

At the airport things got off to an inauspicious start. As we sat in our seats on the United Airlines commuter flight from Sacramento to Los Angeles, where we would change to a direct flight to Charles de Gaulle, we noticed the plane wasn't backing away from the gate. Soon came the announcement of an equipment problem delaying our takeoff. Tony and I realized we weren't going to make the Los Angeles flight to Paris if we continued to sit there.

While others onboard chatted about what was going on, we quickly got up, grabbed our carry-ons (all we ever take), and headed for the United Airlines check-in counter. Because we'd acted so swiftly, the agent was able to get us on a TWA flight just about to depart for St. Louis. From there, we could change to a non-stop TWA flight to Charles de Gaulle, arriving about the same time as we'd originally planned. Like characters on a TV commercial, we ran down the concourse to the TWA boarding gate, our carry-ons in tow. The flight had already boarded but they let us on.

Once off the ground, we praised ourselves. We'd been so much smarter than the other passengers. By the time we left the United Airlines counter with our TWA tickets in hand, those who'd been on the commuter flight had formed a long line behind us. Ah, pride. "Caution, caution," the Buddha would have said, but at that moment we were so pleased with ourselves for deftly averting a disastrous beginning to our special vacation. Several doctors have told us the odds are high that on one of these two TWA flights I picked up the virus from which I have never recovered.

We arrived at our studio apartment on the tiny *Rue du Vieux Colombier* in the sixth arrondissement on the Left Bank. The apartment was much smaller than it had looked in the online pictures. It consisted of a bathroom and a kitchen, each of which could be comfortably occupied by only one person at a time, and a living room. It was furnished with a tiny table and two chairs, a loveseat (a romantic euphemism for a couch that's too small to lie down on), and a double bed in the corner. On the wall opposite the bed sat a bookshelf with a cabinet at the bottom. We found a tiny television set inside, but we had no intention of spending our time in Paris watching TV.

We wandered around that first day, waiting for nightfall so we could sleep and adjust to the new time zone. The next day, I felt awful but assumed it was only jet lag. The day after that, I still felt bad but, refusing to believe it could be anything other than lingering jet lag, suggested we go to a movie. We picked an American film, *Anniversary Party*. Frankly, I just wanted to sit in the dark and try to assess what was going on in my body. While watching the movie I began to realize that I was indeed sick.

Soon thereafter, I developed typical flu symptoms and couldn't get out of bed. After three days, Tony and I reached the same hopeful conclusion: "This is no big deal. We still have eighteen days left in Paris."

After a week, it became: "No big deal, we still have two weeks left in Paris."

". . .we still have ten days left in Paris."

The "days left" dwindled and dwindled.

We developed a routine. In the morning, Tony would go to a *brasserie* and then walk the streets of Paris, returning around noon, always hoping for a change in my condition. Then he'd go out in the afternoon for more walking. Maybe he would take in a museum. He was not enjoying these solo excursions.

During the second week of our stay, I so badly wanted to keep Tony company that I decided one day to tough it out. I insisted we go to see the famous Impressionist collection at the Musée d'Orsay, which was converted from a train station and is known for its soaring interior spaces. The line to get in went around the block. Right then and there, we would have returned to the apartment had I not done my research and known to buy museum passes in the Métro. Under the assumption we'd be museum-hopping together, Tony had bought two passes on our second day in Paris. We were allowed inside immediately.

As soon as I entered the Impressionist gallery, the adrenaline I'd used to get myself there wore off—this excursion had been a mistake. I collapsed into one of the lovely wicker chairs that sit in rows in the middle of the bigger galleries and told Tony to go ahead and enjoy the paintings. He would periodically come back and check on me, asking if we should leave, but I kept telling him to go off and look for a while longer.

As I sat, my eyes lit on a large painting by Claude Monet, *Essai de figure en plein-air: Femme a l'ombrelle tournee vers la droite*. A woman stands in a field, her face shaded by her umbrella. It's painted with a soft, muted palette, yet is somehow wonderfully luminous. I was vaguely aware of musical wicker chairs going on around me—people would sit for a few minutes, get up and be quickly replaced by someone who had been waiting to take the first free chair. I just sat, bathed in the colors and the composition on Monet's canvas. I felt as if he'd painted this young woman in a field to watch over me so I could let Tony experience the museum. But my attempt at keeping him company had failed.

Except to see a doctor, that was the end of going out. My days were spent in bed. Too sick to read, I thought I'd try the little television after all. I was shocked at the poor quality of French programming: every channel had the worst kind of quiz show, featuring contestants who'd been coached to scream on cue, loud-mouthed obnoxious hosts, and the gaudiest of sets. In my naïveté, I was expecting high French culture to emanate from the tube. I gave up in frustration, but as the hours wore on, and I was still bored and restless, I tried TV again. I heard familiar theme music, actors were running around pushing a gurney, and on the screen the word "*Emerges*" appeared. Even with my poor French, I knew this was "ER." I settled in for some televised comfort food, only to find it was dubbed into French. Even movies were dubbed instead of subtitled. So much for that.

I spent most of each day and many a night when I was too sick to sleep listening to the BBC on a short-wave radio Tony bought for me when it was clear I'd be in bed for a while. The BBC had a wonderful array of programs, including clever and funny quiz shows. It became my introduction to our own National Public

Radio (NPR), which I began listening to every day soon after returning to Davis and finding myself bed-bound. When I'm listening to NPR's broadcast of the BBC News and I hear the plummy tones of the very same British voice that came over the short wave radio in our Paris apartment announcing, "You're listening to the BBC World Service," a tinge of sadness passes over me. I'm briefly transported back to that bed on the Left Bank where it all began.

A few days after the trip to the Musée d'Orsay, we decided I should see a doctor. I looked in the yellow pages and found an entry for "the American Hospital." Even though the name suggested home and a refuge for me, the person who answered the phone was just plain rude. When I described my symptoms, she gruffly said, "Well, what do you want *us* to do about it?" It was a harbinger of things to come.

I tried "the British Hospital." The woman who answered the phone only spoke French, but I heard concern and kindness in her voice. She put me on hold while she found a nurse who spoke English. She told me to come right in.

I still shake my head in disbelief when I think of the unnecessary stress we subjected ourselves to getting from our apartment on the Left Bank to the British Hospital in a northern suburb of Paris, and thereafter to a pharmacy in central Paris, and then finally back to the Left Bank. Whew! Typical Californians, we never considered taking a cab. We weren't being cheap; it just didn't cross our minds. We think of cabs as something New Yorkers use. Foolishly, we walked from our apartment to the nearest Métro stop. Two transfers and several staircases later, we found ourselves above ground in an altogether different sort of Paris—the suburbs. Walking along with our map in hand, we made agonizingly slow progress. Even this small excursion was wearing me out.

The doctor thought I simply had the flu. She wrote down my diagnosis as *grippe*—a word that's always made me think of the rhyme for "post-nasal drip" in Adelaide's song from *Guys and Dolls*. She wanted to be sure it didn't turn into a bacterial infection that would ruin our whole vacation, so she gave me a prescription for antibiotics. We trekked back to the Métro and, after another transfer and more stairs, surfaced above ground at the only open pharmacy between the northern suburb and our Left Bank apartment, since it was one of those European days off intriguingly called a bank holiday.

The hospital and pharmacy ordeal is a haze in my mind, although a few vivid memories remain. I recall the hospital staff continually apologizing because, since it was a bank holiday, they had to charge us for the appointment—a whopping $15.00 when converted from francs to dollars. I recall surfacing from the Métro to go to the pharmacy and finding myself face to face with a postcard-picture view of the Arc de Triomphe, the tiniest flash of the Paris we'd hoped for. I also remember the agony I felt as I leaned against the wall in the Métro stairwells, using both hands on the banister to pull my body up step after step. Tony told me, years later, that when he saw me dragging my body up the stairs, he realized how sick I was. That's *his* vivid memory of that day.

Our last week in Paris, I discovered that the French Open was on TV all day long. Tennis was something where language didn't matter. Even I could figure out that "*égalité*" meant "deuce." I made a bed for myself on the floor, close enough to the TV to be able to see the ball being hit over the net, and a love affair was born. I still watch a lot of tennis. I can recite the names of players from all over the world. I love how international tennis is. I love the aesthetics of the game—complexity within seeming simplicity. All a player has to do is get the ball over the net, inside the lines. But within that seeming simplicity lies an array of strategies—physical and mental—that has the feel of a chess game: aces, lobs, volleys, luring your opponent into the net so as to execute a passing shot. As I lay there learning to love watching tennis, it seemed I might be getting better. I was deeply disappointed that our vacation had been ruined, but I was hopeful.

The day before we were scheduled to fly home, I felt I was on the road to recovery.

2

Staying Sick:
This Can't Be Happening to Me

You can argue with the way things are.
You'll lose, but only 100% of the time.
—BYRON KATIE

A WEEK AFTER RETURNING, I HAD A RELAPSE. Then once again, I seemed to get better except, strangely, my voice didn't return. This new whisper of a voice was troublesome because, as a professor, I made my living by talking. With the law school semester starting at the end of August, I talked to the dean in early July about my concerns, but he was confident I'd be fine by then. We agreed not to worry.

Feeling stronger and stronger, in mid-July, I went ahead with plans to go on a ten-day meditation retreat at Spirit Rock Meditation Center, in Marin County, north of San Francisco, about two hours from my home. This was a treasured annual retreat for Buddhist practitioners on the West Coast because the two principal teachers—Joseph Goldstein and Sharon Salzberg—had, along with Jack Kornfield, brought *vipassana* meditation to the United States after intensive training by teachers in Thailand, Burma, and

India. They founded the Insight Meditation Society (IMS) in Barre, Massachusetts, which instantly became a mecca for Americans who wanted to learn to meditate. Some years later, Jack moved to California and, along with other vipassana teachers, founded Spirit Rock. Once a year, Joseph and Sharon, along with other IMS teachers, led a ten-day retreat at Spirit Rock, a retreat so popular that one could only get in through a lottery system. Except for my whisper of a voice, I appeared to be over what my doctor now humorously called "the Parisian Flu." And, besides, one doesn't *need* a voice on a silent retreat. This year, Carol Wilson, Kamala Masters, and Steve Armstrong—all wonderful meditation teachers—accompanied Joseph and Sharon. I thought, "Lucky, lucky me."

It was during this retreat that the Parisian Flu turned from acute to chronic. Eerily, I have it documented, although at the time I didn't know I was describing symptoms that would still be with me years and years later. I'd taken a notebook with me to jot down tidbits from the teachers' talks. It was not intended to be a daily diary, but what was happening to me was too curious not to keep track of. On Monday morning (the third day of the retreat), I wrote, "Woke up feeling sick. Am worried is same stuff again. Determined to stay here even if can only go to Dharma talks."

That night, I wrote, "Feel as if I'm in a stupor. Have this humming, angry pulsating feeling in the body as if I've been up for several nights, not like any other illness I've ever had."

On Tuesday, I wrote, "Definitely sick. What's going on? Very confused."

Determined to stay at the retreat, at one point I wrote, "If one is to be sick and alone, this is as good a place as any." But aside from attending a few talks (there was one each evening) and going to the eating hall once a day for lunch because wiping down the tables afterward was my work meditation, I stayed in my room.

Since the residence halls are up a steep hill from the eating hall, I wrote, "Coming up the hill, I feel like I'm coming up the stairs in the Métro. The flashback is vivid."

Although I felt too sick to sit up and meditate, I tried to follow a basic meditation instruction: Watch the mind. "Worry is arising," I wrote. A neutral, nonattached observation of fact. But I couldn't maintain that meditative perspective for long and so "Worry is arising" was soon followed by an outpouring of troubled thoughts and questions: "Did they read a blood test wrong? . . . I would like to absorb into TV . . . In my room and sad, second-guessing if I should go home to see the doctor. So sad. So sad, especially since I now know the joy of being well."

I didn't go back to work at the end of August in 2001. The dean found someone to cover my classes. I also didn't get to spend time with my new granddaughter, Malia, whose first year of life was going by fast. That fall, my life was spent in bed or at a doctor's office. I entered the phase of the illness in which we needed to rule out every cause that could show up in blood tests, CT scans, MRIs, and other procedures, some of which were completely foreign to me (such as the painful but fascinating appointment where a technician made a videotape of my voice box to be examined for abnormalities).

I had so much blood drawn that we joked with my primary care doctor that at least we'd proven that blood-letting didn't appear to be a cure. I was referred to half a dozen specialists. All I could tell them was that I had flu-like symptoms without the fever; an extremely hoarse voice; eighteen pounds of weight loss; and a fatigue so devastating that, no matter how small the waiting-room chair, I tried to turn it into a bed.

In the end, I saw three infectious disease doctors, two ENT specialists, a rheumatologist, an endocrinologist, a gastroenterologist, a neurologist, a cardiologist, and (on my own) two acupuncturists.

Each ran his or her own battery of tests. Even though I was never referred to an oncologist, I still found myself at a cancer center because the endocrinologist wanted to test my adrenal function using an infusion test that could only be performed at the clinic where cancer patients received chemotherapy. I met some brave people that day.

The testing and physical exams indicated that nothing was wrong with me. So in the spring of 2002, I dragged myself back to the law school twice a week to teach a class that met for ninety minutes each session. I went back to work mainly because I simply could not and would not believe I wasn't going to get better. Everyone I saw at work assumed I'd finally recovered. After all, I didn't look sick to them. They would stop me in the hall to chat, seemingly unaware that I was leaning against the wall to keep from falling over.

I continued to work part-time for two and a half years, sometimes going to the law school twice a week, sometimes three times a week, depending on the class schedule. Even though Tony worked in another town, he tried to arrange his schedule so he could drive me the ten minutes from our house to the law school and pick me up after my class. I was too sick to drive myself ten minutes to work, yet I'd teach a class that sometimes lasted an hour and a half.

It's easy to look back and see what a mistake it was to continue working while sick—it probably worsened my condition—but many people who have contracted a chronic illness have done the same. First, there's the financial need to keep working. Second, there's the utter disbelief that this is happening to you (reinforced by people telling you that you look just fine—people who don't see you collapse on the bed as soon as you get home). Each morning, you expect to wake up *not feeling sick* even though for weeks and then months—and then years—that has never been the case.

It's just so hard to, first, truly recognize that you're chronically ill and, second, to accept that this illness is going to require you to change your plans for life in ways you never imagined, not the least of which is giving up the profession you loved and worked so hard to build.

I had to come up with secret coping mechanisms to make it through my part-time workday. For the first time in twenty years, I took a chair into the classroom and taught while sitting down. The noise made by lively chatting students, as many as eighty at a time, was so jarring to my sick body that I wore ear plugs as I entered the room, then discretely removed them as the students quieted down for me to begin talking. I concocted a method to keep students from coming to my office because, once I was in there with them, I lost the ability to control the length of the interaction. If someone approached me after class and another class was following mine in the same room, I'd find an empty classroom and sit down there with the student. That way, when I felt I'd answered his or her questions, I could stand up and end the conversation.

I even had a secret coping technique I didn't tell Tony about because it felt too deviant. My office wasn't close to a bathroom. Not only was I too sick to walk to the bathroom on the other side of the building, but doing so would risk running into colleagues who might (with the best of intentions) want to engage me in conversation while standing in the hallway. Avoiding those encounters was among my highest priorities. So I found an old thermos and took it to my office. I peed into it, screwed the lid on tightly, put it in my bag, and took it home to empty and wash out.

Those who have no choice but to go to work while sick all have such secret coping mechanisms. At first, I felt humiliated having to use subterfuges and to undergo such indignity just to relieve myself. I blamed myself for my life having brought me to this sorry state. After a while, the self-loathing shifted to a defiant but ugly cynicism: healthy people be damned; this is what I'm doing, so shove it if you don't approve. Fortunately, the cynicism gave way to compassion for myself. If nothing else, peeing into a thermos was no easy feat: I was professionally dressed for class, pantyhose and all.

I never told the students I was sick (although some of them figured it out). However, being sick, I was unable to be anyone other than my unadorned self in the classroom. It became easy to admit that I didn't have all the answers, and I felt a new compassion both for people caught up in the legal system and for students facing struggles in their own lives. Sitting in a chair, speaking in such a weak voice that students sometimes had to ask me to repeat myself, I received the highest teaching evaluations in my twenty years on the job. And yet, I had to let it all go. When you are as chronically ill as I am, you have to make some very hard choices. Ironically, people may think you're giving up, when in fact you are simply giving in to the reality of your new life.

For me, that reality meant having the symptoms that accompany a severe flu, including the dazed sick feeling and low-grade headache, but without the fever, the sore throat, and the cough. To imagine it, multiply the extreme fatigue of a flu by an order of magnitude. Add in a heart pounding with the kind of wired, oppressive fatigue that healthy people associate with severe jet lag, making it hard to concentrate or even watch TV—let alone to nap or even sleep at night.

Part of the reality of chronic debilitating illness is continually trying to figure out why you are so sick—and never getting a definitive answer. If being labeled with an acronym could cure me, I'd be in great shape. Since getting sick in Paris, I've been diagnosed with a laundry list of diseases and conditions: CFS (aka CFIDS, ME), PVS, VICD, OI, and POTS. (If you'd like to know what these letters and various diagnoses mean, see the box on pages 15–17.)

In the end, though, all we really know is this: I got sick on a trip to Paris and I never got well. But I also began a journey into the depths of the Buddha's teaching. I needed to learn how to be sick.

How do you name my illness?
Let me count the ways.

Chronic Fatigue Syndrome. "CFS is a 'garbage pail' diagnosis," an infectious disease specialist told Tony and me. He said doctors use it when it's clear that a patient is sick but standard medical tests have failed to pinpoint the cause. CFS has become the default diagnosis given to me. It's what doctors write down on forms. (The medical slang "garbage pail" is rejected by all the major CFS experts whose tireless efforts to solve the mystery of symptoms that have been collectively labeled "CFS" have given hope to millions saddled with this diagnosis.)

Chronic Fatigue and Immune Dysfunction Syndrome. CFIDS is an alternative name given to CFS, partially in an attempt to have it taken seriously and partially because a subset of CFS patients appear to have an overactive immune system that produces flu-like symptoms as the body remains in a perpetual state of "sickness response."

Myalgic Encephomyalitis. ME is the name given to CFS in almost every country but the United States. Its literal translation would be "muscle pain and brain inflammation," but it's as non-descriptive of what sufferers experience as is the phrase Chronic Fatigue Syndrome—although being diagnosed with ME avoids being simplistically labeled as someone who is just complaining about being tired. CFS, CFIDS, and ME are synonymous and purport to describe the same illness. But I've met dozens of people on the Internet who have been given one of these diagnoses and none of us have identical symptoms. Some have chronic sore throats and swollen lymph glands. Others (like me) do not, but suffer from an unremitting flu-like malaise. Some experience cognitive impairment, including difficulty processing information, forgetfulness, and an inability to form sentences properly. Others (like me) do not, except to the extent that the flu-like symptoms make it hard to concentrate. Some suffer from muscle and joint pain. Others (like me) do not. The only symptom that those with this diagnosis share is "fatigue" (which is a feature of almost every illness, from the common cold to cancer). And even this symptom ranges from a fatigue that sets in only after a person is active, to an ever-present bone-crushing fatigue that prevents a person from ever straying far from the bed. I'm convinced that CFS encompasses several discrete illnesses and that until the general medical community recognizes this, little progress will be made in finding a cause or a cure.

Post-Viral Syndrome. A few decades ago, the Centers for Disease Control (the CDC) rejected the name PVS in favor of CFS. Some doctors still use the name Post-Viral Syndrome and did so with me, especially in the first two years following the "Parisian Flu."

Viral Induced Central Nervous System Dysfunction. VICD is a fairly recent designation, used to describe a subset of CFS patients whose blood work indicates there may be a reactivation of herpes viruses that usually lay dormant in the body after their acute childhood phases. My blood work suggests that I fit this subset, although antivirals haven't helped me. The theory is that an acute infection—in my case, the "Parisian Flu"—triggers a reactivation of the viruses, causing the immune system to become engaged in a constant low-grade war against them.

Orthostatic Intolerance and *Postural Tachycardia Syndrome.* These two diagnoses refer to poor blood circulation, which makes it difficult to maintain a standing position. They are thought to be results of whatever is wrong with me as opposed to the cause.

Accepting Pain

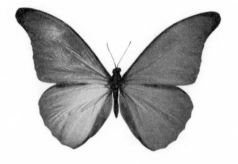

3

The Buddha Tells It Like It Is

To go into the dark with a light is to know the light.
To know the dark, go dark. Go without sight
and find that the dark, too, blooms and sings,
and is traveled by dark feet and dark wings.

—WENDELL BERRY

AFTER A LONG AND WINDING JOURNEY OF DISCOVERY with many ups and downs, the Buddha, an ordinary human being like you and me, sat down under a tree for a long time, and then he attained enlightenment—also known as liberation, freedom, or awakening. At first he wasn't sure if he could find the words to share his discovery, but eventually he gave his first teaching in the form of the Four Noble Truths. Buddhism—what Buddhists call the Dharma, which simply means "teachings"—was born.

Many people will tell you they know the first noble truth, but their usual rendering, "Life is suffering," is responsible for a lot of misunderstanding about what the Buddha taught. In offering us the first noble truth, the Buddha was not making a negative pronouncement. If so, it's hard to imagine why he would have called it "noble."

"Life is suffering" is misleading for at least two reasons. First, the Buddha used an ancient Indian language similar to Sanskrit called Pali, and the word he used in Pali for the first noble truth, *dukkha*, is difficult to translate. *Dukkha* is too multifaceted and nuanced a term to be captured in the one-word translation "suffering." And second, the fact of dukkha in our lives doesn't mean that life is *only* dukkha.

To capture the essence of what the Buddha meant by the presence of dukkha in our lives, it's helpful to keep other possible translations of this key word in mind: unsatisfactoriness (that is, dissatisfaction with the circumstances of our life), anguish, stress, discomfort, dis-ease, to name just a few. Dukkha is a term worth becoming familiar with, especially when exploring how to be sick. When I first encountered the various translations for dukkha, they resonated powerfully for me. Finally, someone was describing this life in a way that fit a good portion of my experience, both physical and mental: stress, discomfort, unsatisfactoriness. What a relief to know it wasn't just *me*, or wasn't just *my* life!

The feeling that the Buddha understood the pain of my life allowed me to start the day-to-day work of accepting that dukkha is present for all beings. Even in the darkest early days of the illness, when I didn't understand what was happening to me (was I dying?), I always had the first noble truth propping me up, telling me, "You know this is the way it is. You were born and so are subject to change, disease, and ultimately death. It happens differently for each person. This is one of the ways it's happening to you."

I'll never forget listening to Spirit Rock teacher John Travis giving a talk on a ten-day retreat. He suddenly stopped talking and slowly scanned the room, making eye contact with every single one of us. Then he very gently said, "I know you. We all know each other. We've all had our hearts broken by the relentless search to avoid suffering." I would only add that this relentless search just brings more suffering because dukkha is an aspect of existence for all living beings born into this world.

The first noble truth—the fact of dukkha—helps me accept being sick because that fact tells me my life is as it should be. "Our life is always all right," says Zen teacher Charlotte Joko Beck. "There's nothing wrong with it. Even if we have horrendous problems, it's just our life."

Joko Beck points out that the second part of the word *suffer* (*-fer*) is from the Latin verb *ferre* which means "to bear" and that the first part (*suf-*) is from *sub*, meaning "under." Taking this view, dukkha is not about life bearing down on us from the *outside*, but instead dukkha is an internal phenomenon of bearing life up from underneath. Joko Beck writes:

> So there are two kinds of suffering. One is when we feel we're being pressed down; as though suffering is coming at us from without, as though we're receiving something that's making us suffer. The other kind of suffering is being under, just bearing it, just *being* it.

Just "being" life as it is for me has meant ending my professional career years before I expected to, being house-bound and even bed-bound much of the time, feeling continually sick in the body, and not being able to socialize very often. Using Joko Beck's teaching, I was able to use these facts that make up my life as a starting point. I began to bow down to these facts, to accept them, to *be* them. And then from there, I looked around to see what life had to offer.

And I found a lot.

The End of Suffering

As I said above, the Buddha didn't say that life is *only* suffering, stressful, unsatisfactory. He simply taught that dukkha is present in the life of all beings. Years ago, a law student told me that Buddhism was a pessimistic religion. When I asked him why he thought that, he said, "Well, its first noble truth is: Life sucks." In trying to explain to him why that was not a valid translation of the Buddha's teaching, a shift occurred in how I thought of the first noble truth. Yes, it's true that life brings with it a considerable share of suffering and stress, but happiness and joy are also available to us. The Buddha expressed this by describing life as the realm of the ten thousand joys and the ten thousand sorrows. Buddhist teachers focus on those ten thousand sorrows because our inability to see the truth of dukkha in our lives only increases it.

The Buddha said he taught dukkha and the end of dukkha. Before we get into practices that have helped me on the path to the "end of dukkha," we need to be very clear about the truth of dukkha itself, so we can understand what the "end of dukkha" might mean. It's fruitless to begin the quest for the end of dukkha until we see that our life is just as it should be—dukkha and all. Do you know a single person, healthy or sick in body, who has not experienced suffering, unsatisfactoriness, anguish, stress, discomfort, dis-ease?

When I taught a class in Tort Law, we spent several weeks studying damages available to plaintiffs in a civil action. "Specials" are those damages for which plaintiff has a receipt: $1,000 for an MRI, for instance. "Generals" are referred to as plaintiff's "pain and suffering." No receipts here—the jury is simply asked to put a monetary value on this intangible damage. "Pain and suffering" is a stock phrase in the legal profession. Based on my Buddhist training, I decided to break down this category of damages into "bodily pain and mental suffering" simply because I thought it would help students understand the jury's task better. The distinction applies here too, because when the Buddha talked about the "end of dukkha," he wasn't referring to putting an end to bodily pain, which is an inescapable part of the human condition. The Buddha was talking about the end of *suffering in the mind*—the theme of the rest of this book.

After the first noble truth points to the pervasiveness of suffering, the remaining truths start us down the road of what to do about it, how to work on the end of suffering in the mind. The second noble truth says that the reason for dukkha—which we're thinking of as *mental* suffering, stress, anguish—is the truth of *tanha*. The literal translation of *tanha* is "thirst," a concept not far from the popular conception of the second noble truth—that the origin of suffering is desire. I think of *tanha* as the seemingly ever-present mental states of "want" and "don't want" in our lives. We want pleasant experiences; we don't want unpleasant ones.

The third noble truth proclaims the good news that the end of dukkha is possible. And in the fourth noble truth, the Buddha sets out the lesson plan to accomplish this. That lesson plan is contained in the Eightfold Path. By following the Eightfold Path, we can learn to cultivate the wholesome and joyful mind states I referred to above. With the end of dukkha comes "enlightenment," "awakening," "liberation," "freedom," or "unbinding"—I recommend you pick the translation that resonates best with you.

We may not be able to complete the lesson plan of the Eightfold Path during our lifetime. That is, we may not become fully enlightened beings, but that glimpse of awakening, that moment of liberation, that taste of freedom is available to us all—and can take us a long way toward easing our experience of dukkha.

4

The Universal Law of Impermanence

Better a single day of life
seeing the reality of arising and passing away
than a hundred years of existence remaining blind to it.
—THE BUDDHA

ENDING DUKKHA IN THE MIND includes understanding what the Buddha called the "three marks of existence." We have already been discussing the first mark: the fact of dukkha in our lives. The other two are impermanence (*anicca*) and no-self (*anatta*). When the Buddha began explaining these characteristics of our existence, he began with impermanence. It is a universal law, recognized in other spiritual traditions and in science as common to the life of every living being.

At a Spirit Rock retreat in the late 1990s, Joseph Goldstein gave what has come to be my favorite description of anicca as I experience it in everyday life: "Anything can happen at any time."

Initially, I reacted to his statement the same way I reacted when I first heard *anicca* translated from the Pali as "Everything is impermanent." I thought, "Yeah, tell me something I *don't* know." But when I didn't recover my health, I began to deeply contemplate the meaning of "anything can happen at any time"—like getting sick and not getting better, like having to give up my profession, like rarely being able to leave the house. Yes, anything *can* happen at any time. Life is impermanent, uncertain, unpredictable, ever-changing.

How are we to find any solace in this universal law? The great Zen master Dogen offers a clue:

> Without the bitterest cold that penetrates to the very bone, how can plum blossoms send forth their fragrance all over the universe?

When we begin to see the truth of anicca, there's a tendency to focus on "the bitterest cold that penetrates to the very bone" phrase in Dogen's words. Having had to give up my profession still feels like that on some days. The challenge becomes finding the fragrance sent forth by those plum blossoms. Without the bitter cold of giving up my profession, I wouldn't have the fragrance of Mozart and Beethoven wafting through my bedroom. (Of course, I *could* have enjoyed that fragrance before I got sick, but the fact is, I didn't.) Without the bitter cold of having to stay in bed most of the day, I wouldn't be so attuned to the changing seasons; I never realized they are on view right outside my bedroom window. I return to Dogen's verse over and over for inspiration.

The writings of the Vietnamese Zen master Thich Nhat Hanh have also helped me see the beauty inherent in the fact of imper-manence. In his biography of the Buddha, *Old Path White Clouds*, Thich Nhat Hanh points out that impermanence is the very con-dition necessary for life. Without it, nothing could grow or develop. A grain of rice could not grow into a rice plant; a child could not grow into an adult. There are so many ways in which I've "grown" only because of this illness, from my newfound love of classical music, to a heightened compassion for the chronically ill and their caregivers, to an appreciation for the hard-working people who go unnoticed but keep our infrastructure running. (I see them from my house—delivering mail, climbing power poles, cleaning the streets—whether it's over 100 degrees out or pouring rain.)

Weather Practice

Buddhist teachers use any number of English words to translate *anicca:* impermanence, change, unpredictability, uncertainty. All are characteristics common to existence—animate and inanimate. Two of those words, *uncertainty* and *unpredictability*, can be a source of a great deal of anxiety and suffering for us because we desire just the opposite: security and assurance. Here, I offer a practice that addresses these two aspects of impermanence. I call it "weather practice"; it was inspired by, of all things, the 2005 movie *The Weather Man*, starring Nicolas Cage as a character named Dave Spritz.

Dave is adrift in life, even though he has a steady job as the weatherman for a Chicago TV station. In reality, he's just a "weather reader," dependent on a meteorologist to tell him what to say. When the meteorologist gives him a forecast with an eighteen-degree variance, Dave complains that he needs something more concrete. The meteorologist responds, "Dave, it's random. We do our best." One day the meteorologist preps Dave for his TV spot by saying, "We might see some snow, but it might shift south and miss us." When Dave protests that the viewers will want a more certain forecast than that, the meteorologist tells him that predicting the weather is a guess. "It's wind, man," he says. "It blows all over the place."

I found this inspiring and very useful. When life's uncertainty and unpredictability throw me for a loop, I like to say to Tony:

"Here it is again, life and the weather. Just wind, man, blowing all over the place." Then returning to the verse from Dogen, I remind myself that the wind that's blowing the bitterest cold at me may be setting the stage for something joyful to follow.

I work on treating thoughts and moods as wind, blowing into the mind and blowing out. We can't control what thoughts arise in the mind. (Telling yourself not to think about whether you'll feel well enough to join the family for dinner is almost a guarantee that it's exactly what you *will* think about!) And moods are as uncontrollable as thoughts. Blue moods arise uninvited, as does fear or anxiety. By working with this wind metaphor, I can hold painful thoughts and blue moods more lightly, knowing they'll blow on through soon—after all, that's what they do.

One night, I felt so sick I wanted to throw out all the work I'd done on this book. Dark thoughts. A blue mood. My eyes welled up with tears. But instead of those tears turning into sobs, I took a deep breath and began the weather practice, remembering that thoughts and moods blow all over the place and that if I just waited, these particular ones would blow on through. And they did.

When it became clear that the Parisian Flu had settled into a chronic illness, Tony and I began to consider if it was feasible for him to go on a retreat for an entire month during which he'd be out of contact with me unless I called with an emergency. I badly wanted him to go because I saw it as a way I could feel like a caregiver for him. He went for the first time in 2005 and each February thereafter. The retreat became a major annual event for him. The preparations he made ahead of time were like those that people make who are in the path of a coming hurricane. He brought a month of supplies into the house. He filled the freezer with food he'd cooked ahead of time. He set up people in town for me to contact if I needed help. My promise to him was to be extra careful in everything I did and to call him home if I needed him.

The forecast inside our house for February 2009 called for calm weather despite my illness. But at 9:00 A.M., two days after Tony left, things changed in a split second. One moment I was at the top of the two steps that lead down to our bedroom—the next moment I was writhing in pain on the bedroom floor, having slipped down the steps and landed on my right ankle.

When the pain began to subside, I pulled myself up on the bed and went straight to my laptop to research the only question on my mind: Was I going to have to go to the doctor? Medical appointments can be an ordeal for the chronically ill—the roundtrip drive, the possibility of a long wait, the energy it takes to effectively communicate with the doctor. It's so much easier to have a caregiver along. When I go to the doctor, Tony drives me, stands in line to check in for me, and accompanies me to the examining room. I never schedule medical appointments during February.

Despite the rapidly increasing swelling and discoloration on my ankle, my Internet research convinced me that I only needed to go to the doctor if I still couldn't put weight on it in twenty-four hours. So I waited. And when I needed to go somewhere off the bed, I crawled. Our dog, Rusty, was delighted to see this. He acted like I'd finally seen the light and was joining his species. This appeared to be a cause for great celebration on his part, so my challenge became to make sure that in his exuberance he didn't step on my right foot.

That first day, as I lay in pain on the bed, I thought of the meteorologist's comment to Dave the weather reader: "Dave, it's random. We do our best." Tony and I had indeed done our best to prepare for a calm February, but as we all discover again and again anything can happen at any time. We can take precautions, but predicting the future is as futile as predicting which way the wind will blow.

The next morning, when I still couldn't put weight on my right foot, our friend Richard took me to the doctor. Diagnosis: fractured fibula. The forecast: No weight bearing on it for several weeks; a cast so heavy that it took all my energy to move my leg; crutches and crawling to get around. I toughed it out for one more day. Even with people offering to help, the injury on top of the illness proved to be too much. One or the other I could have handled alone, but not both. I knew I needed to call Tony home when, before going to sleep for the night, it took me ten minutes to make the roundtrip to a bathroom that's only footsteps from the bed. As I lay back on the bed in exhaustion, I realized that the light over the bathroom sink was still on—a light that shines right in my eyes. I had no choice but to start the process of getting to the bathroom all over again.

So Tony came home four days into his treasured month-long retreat and, for a month, traded his caregiver role for that of nursemaid. Life and the weather—one moment it's calm and the next moment a nasty storm has blown in.

Weather practice is a powerful reminder of the fleeting nature of experience, how each moment arises and passes as quickly as a weather pattern. A week after I fell, I went to see an orthopedic surgeon. My regular doctor arranged the consult in case I needed surgery to insert a plate and pins. A resident came in the examining room first. Looking at the x-rays, he said that, given the nature of the break and the damage to the ligaments, I might very well need surgery to stabilize the area. He left the room to report his findings to the orthopedic surgeon—and dark storm clouds gathered as Tony and I contemplated the effect on my illness if I had to go through surgery. Expecting heavy rain to accompany the surgeon into the room, he walked in and immediately said, "Surgery? No, no, no! The area is stable. You just need to stay off the ankle as long as it hurts and get physical therapy to regain your range of motion." In a flash, the sun had burst through the clouds. Tony and I were elated.

But a half-hour later, as I lay on the bed trying to nap, a cold dense fog settled in as I thought, "What does it matter that the surgeon gave us such good news. Even when I can walk normally again, I'll still be sick and bed-bound most of the day and Tony, despite all this extra care he's giving me, still won't have my company out there in the world." In a little over an hour, I'd experienced dark storm clouds, the threat of rain, the sun bursting through instead, and now a cold dense fog. Recognizing the fleeting nature of each moment, I was able to smile and the final verse of the *Diamond Sutra* came to mind:

> Thus shall you think of all this fleeting world:
> A star at dawn, a bubble in a stream;
> A flash of lightning in a summer cloud,
> A flickering lamp, a phantom, and a dream.

I knew it wouldn't be long before the sun would burn off that cold dense fog and I'd smell the fragrance of Dogen's plum blossoms.

Broken-Glass Practice

Finally, to help me live gracefully with the truth of uncertainty and unpredictability, I follow what I call "broken-glass practice." This practice was inspired by a passage in *Food for the Heart*, a collection of the teachings of the Thai Buddhist monk Ajahn Chah. He trained many Westerners at his remote forest monastery and has had a strong influence on the shape that Buddhism of south Asia has taken in the West. As we shall see in more detail later, he offers powerful teachings on equanimity, which is often described as the ability to weather life's ups and downs with a calm and even-tempered mind.

Here is Ajahn Chah talking about a glass:

> You say, "Don't break my glass!" Can you prevent something that's breakable from breaking? It will break sooner or later. If you don't break it, someone else will. If someone else doesn't break it, one of the chickens will! . . . Penetrating the truth of these things, [we see] that this glass is already broken. . . . [the Buddha] saw the broken glass within the unbroken one. Whenever you use this glass, you should reflect that it's already broken. Whenever its time is up, it will break. Use the glass, look after it, until the day when it slips out of your hand and shatters. No problem. Why not? Because you saw its brokenness before it broke!

I use broken-glass practice all the time. The Buddha taught that all that arises is subject to change, decay, and dissolution. So when Tony or I break something, or the power goes off, or the phone line goes dead because the neighborhood squirrels have been chewing on the wires again, we try to laugh and say, "Ah, it was already broken."

As a metaphor, broken-glass practice has helped me accept one of the consequences of being sick that my online wanderings tell me would show up on the "top ten most difficult adjustments" list of anyone who is chronically ill: The very activities that bring us the greatest joy are also the activities that make our condition worse. This was a bitter pill for me to swallow; it still is sometimes.

These activities include everything from holiday dinners to special events, such as weddings. Having to sit upright for extended periods, trying to focus on a conversation while the room is full of noise, not feeling we can leave (or not having the means to leave) even though our bodies are crying out for us to lie down, are but a few of the features of these activities that exacerbate the symptoms of the chronically ill. Even people who are in good health find these gatherings to be exhausting and may need a day or two to recover, so it's not surprising that they can have such a devastating effect on those who are already sick.

At the end of this book is a guide that lists several practices that can help us adjust to this most difficult aspect of impermanence— this unexpected change to our lives that suddenly keeps us from participating in activities that we had counted among our greatest joys. Broken-glass practice can be particularly helpful here. I find comfort in contemplating that my ability to participate in these activities was already broken, in the sense that this change in my life will befall everyone at some point and quite possibly by surprise. This is simply how and when it happened to me.

Then I reflect on impermanence—the fact that every aspect of my life is uncertain, unpredictable, and in constant flux. Finally, like Ajahn Chah, I look after each moment, cherishing what I still *can* do, aware that everything could change in an instant.

5

Who Is Sick?

What I am, as system theorists have helped me see,
is a "flow-through." I am a flow-through
of matter, energy, and information.

—JOANNA MACY

Before getting sick, I had the good fortune of attending several retreats at Spirit Rock co-led by the Theravadan teacher Kamala Masters. At a retreat in 2000, she told us a story about her root teacher, Munindra-ji, who lived in India.

Munindra-ji had always wanted to see the Buddhist sacred sites. He was getting quite old, so Kamala traveled to India with some friends to take him to some of the sites. One day, they were waiting in a train station. The train was five hours late. It was blazing hot. They had no food. There were no restrooms. The track where they were to catch the train kept changing, so they had to keep getting up and moving. Munindra-ji would sit down in each new location and rest his head on his arm. He looked so frail that Kamala began to worry about how he was holding up, especially since she and her friends were barely coping with the conditions. She finally asked him if he was all right. He replied, "There is heat here, but I am not hot. There is hunger here, but I am not hungry. There is irritation here, but I am not irritated."

I recalled Kamala's story one day as I lay in bed after becoming sick, so I silently said, "There is sickness here, but I am not sick." The statement made no sense to me. But, inspired by the story, I persevered, repeating over and over "There is sickness here, but I am not sick . . . There is sickness here, but I am not sick." After a few minutes, I realized, "Of course! There is sickness in the body, but *I* am not sick!"

It was a revelation and a source of great comfort. After a time, however, I decided to investigate more deeply. When I did, this question arose, "Who is this 'I' who isn't sick?" This question led me to consider *anatta* or "no fixed and unchanging self." The Buddha's teaching on no-fixed-self was (and still is) revolutionary. It is the principal way in which he broke from the religion of his birth, Hinduism. Of course, to communicate with others, we have to use conventional terminology such as "I Me Mine" (to borrow from the title of the George Harrison song on the *Let It Be* album). If I'm unwilling to use the term "Toni Bernhard" I can't get a driver's license or a disability check. And, as this very paragraph illustrates, I'll continue to use self-referential terms in this book. But I can use the word "I" and, even as the word emerges from the mind, still contemplate questions such as: "Who am I? What is Toni Bernhard? Is Toni Bernhard a solid physical and mental entity with an inherent self-existence or is Toni Bernhard a label attached to an ever-changing constellation of qualities?" This is worth investigating, for all of us.

We all have a vague or even specific sense of "I am." It is this sense that leads the mind to imagine the existence of a permanent, unchanging self or soul around which our whole life revolves. Joseph Goldstein and Jack Kornfield express this beautifully in *Seeking the Heart of Wisdom:*

Just as we condition our bodies in different ways through exercise or lack of it, so we also condition our minds. Every mind state, thought, or emotion that we experience repeatedly becomes stronger and more habituated. Who we are as personalities is a collection of all the tendencies of mind that have developed, the particular energy configurations we have cultivated.

Think of who you were ten years ago. The part of your personality that seems to be consistent from then until now results, not from any permanent entity carrying over from one moment to the next, but from each moment being conditioned by the previous one. You cannot identify a permanent self that has carried over from ten years ago until now. "I" is a thought and a feeling, held on to so resolutely that the experience of a fixed person appears to be real.

Think of a bicycle. It's just a temporary assemblage of steel, plastic, and human intelligence in a particular combination we conveniently designate "bicycle." There is no inherent "bike-ness." It is the same with humans. There is no immutable, unchanging personality ("Toni Bernhard") that exists as an entity separate from the arising and passing of physical and mental activity—activity that is conditioned by preceding causes. No phenomenon—mental or physical—exists separate and independent from the conditions that give rise to it. This view is in contrast to religions that posit an immutable, eternal being or spiritual essence that is beyond cause and effect. As Steven Collins says in *Selfless Persons*, "there is nothing more to the 'person' but a temporary assemblage of parts."

Contemplating the truth of no-fixed-self has helped me tremendously since I became chronically ill. Haven't we all at some time thought, "If I could only get away from myself!" Intuitively, we know what a relief it would be to take I Me Mine out of the equation. (George Harrison's voice gently reminds us of the unremitting presence of "selfing" when he sings, "Even those tears, *I-me-mine, I-me-mine, I-me-mine*.") Experiencing no-self lifts a burden and brings a sense of spaciousness and freedom to everyday life.

Seeing impermanence can help us experience no-self. Joseph Goldstein said during a retreat I attended that the mind and the body feel substantial, set, and solid, but if we watch carefully, there's nothing to hold on to. "Where's the mood you were in five minutes ago?" he asked. "Where's the thought of a few seconds ago? Where's that expert knowing self of two hours ago?" He suggested the answer was, "Gone!" When I contemplated his words, I saw that mood, that thought, that expert as momentary arisings in the mind.

Joseph went on to explain that we take these momentary arisings and string them together and soon they feel like something solid. Again, I contemplated this. "Ah, yes," I thought. "I string my thoughts together and then feel like the fixed entity: Toni Bernhard." He asked us to see if we could control this fixed entity by issuing commands such as "Let me only have pleasant moods!" or "Let me not have this aching back!" I tried but could not get the mind or the body to obey these commands. What happens in life arises out of conditions, not from a "me" in control.

This teaching can be disturbing to people, but I hope that, like me, you find it liberating. I like to purposefully think, "I am Toni Bernhard" and then contemplate if this is true. People *call* me "Toni Bernhard" and I respond when they do. (I get up from the waiting-room chair at the doctor's office when those two words are called out!) But I can find no fixed, unchanging, permanent entity. There is no Toni Bernhard. And that's fine. Life is a process and will take whatever course it takes.

Contemplating the perennial question "Who Am I?" can also help us experience "no self." This question is a tool used by Western philosophers and Eastern mystics alike, although their answers to the question may differ. For instance, in *The Only Dance There Is*, spiritual teacher Ram Dass discusses the difference in the Western and Eastern approaches to this question, comparing Descartes' "I think, therefore I am" with the more anatta-flavored formulation, "I think, but I am not my thoughts."

While in India in 1967, Richard Alpert became a disciple of the Hindu sage Neem Karoli Baba, who gave him the name Ram Dass. Neem Karoli Baba didn't give formal discourses. He told stories and sometimes spoke only a few words to a disciple before sending him or her away. Many years ago, I read an interview with Ram Dass in which he said that when he was preparing to return to the U.S., he asked Neem Karoli Baba what teaching he should take home with him. The sage told him to just keep asking the question, "Who Am I?" as he went about his daily activities. Zen masters also use this question as a koan, giving it to students to contemplate.

So, *Who am I?*

Am I my body?

No. If I were my body, it would obey the command not to be sick.

Am I my mind?

No. If I were my mind, it would obey the command not to worry about things.

Who am I?

In the epigraph that heads this chapter, Joanna Macy answers the question like this, "I am a flow-through of matter, energy, and information." This may not be your answer, but keeping the question in the mind helps break down the sense of a solid, permanent self that leads to fixed (and limiting) identities such as "I am a sick person" or "I am a caregiver for a sick person." Shedding these fixed identities opens possibilities for seeing the world with new eyes. The answer to "Who Am I?" remains a mystery to me—and

I'm content with that. Mysteries are compelling and intriguing and, in this case, also quite liberating.

Sky-Gazing Practice

To help me experience "no self," I use a practice called "sky-gazing" from the Dzogchen tradition of Tibetan Buddhism. I lie down in my backyard, look up at the sky, and relax my gaze. After a while, the experience takes on an openness and a spaciousness. All notions of a separate self—in body or in mind—dissolve. There may be a sound or a sensation of a breeze going by or a thought arising, but it is all just energy, flowing through. Although this spaciousness may last only a few seconds, in those seconds, there's no Toni Bernhard.

Even when the illusion of Toni Bernhard re-emerges as a solid, separate entity (as it always eventually does!), those few seconds without it were so liberating that a serene glow stays with me for a while. Gradually, the glow fades and identities start piling on: former dean and law professor, wife, mother, dog-owner, sick person. But I can always sky-gaze again.

I use a variation of sky-gazing while lying in bed, especially at night when I'm unable to sleep due to symptoms of the illness. I close my eyes and consciously switch my focus away from awareness of unpleasant bodily sensations by letting my pupils roll upward toward the top of my head. This signals that I've made a shift in consciousness that's the equivalent of sky-gazing. Soon, identities start peeling away, including the identity "sick person." The body is experienced as pulsating matter, teeming with energy. The mind is experienced as a conduit for information that flows in and flows out.

"No self, no problem," a popular Buddhist saying goes. And everything is okay just as it is—sickness and all.

Finding Joy and Love

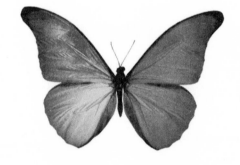

6

Finding Joy in the Life You Can No Longer Lead

We should find perfect existence through imperfect existence.

—SHUNRYU SUZUKI

A S WITH MANY ORAL TRADITIONS that transmit their spiritual teachings from generation to generation by word of mouth, the Buddha's teachings were often passed down in lists—like the Four Noble Truths and the Eightfold Path, which many people have heard of who've never studied any Buddhism. Lists work because they make the teachings easier to commit to memory. Nevertheless, Buddhists like to joke about both the staggering number of lists and the number of concepts that appear on multiple lists. No matter which list we use to enter the teachings, it won't be long before we reach the Buddha's core teaching: the fact of suffering in our lives and the practices that can lead to the end of that suffering through awakening, liberation, freedom.

For me, the sweetest list is the four *brahma viharas*, often translated as the four "sublime states." I love the dictionary definition of sublime: "so awe-inspiringly beautiful as to seem heavenly." Simply put, these are mental states we would be wise to cultivate because they are the dwelling place of the enlightened or awakened mind. Indeed, in Pali, *vihara* also means "dwelling place."

The four brahma viharas are:

> *Metta*—loving-kindness; wishing well to others and to
> ourselves
> *Karuna*—compassion; reaching out to those who are
> suffering, including ourselves
> *Mudita*—sympathetic joy; joy in the joy of others
> *Upekkha*—equanimity; a mind that is at peace in all
> circumstances.

Neem Karoli Baba often told his disciples, "Don't throw anyone out of your heart"—and "anyone" would, of course, include ourselves. This one powerful sentence encompasses all four sublime states, and I would only temper his words by invoking the same intention as the Zen teacher Robert Aitken does when he recites the Buddhist precepts, its code of ethical conduct. He begins the recitation with: "I undertake the practice of . . ." I like this because words like "don't" or "always" can set us up for failure. I won't always be able to cultivate the four sublime states, but I vow to undertake the practice of cultivating them—the practice of not throwing anyone out of my heart.

Let's start our exploration of these sublime states by considering sympathetic joy and take up the other three after that. Cultivating *joy in the joy of others* has been central to coming to terms with the life I can no longer lead. Without this, I'd be steeped in envy. Because our activities are so limited, it's hard for the chronically ill to avoid feeling envy for all those people just living their lives as they always have. Some of us must stay at home, unable to join family and friends when they go to a movie or take a bike ride or attend weddings and other special events or go on vacation or even dash out to the store for a quart of milk. Even those who are not house-bound have to pace themselves carefully and so, for example, cannot always spontaneously visit or go out for a meal with family and friends. These limitations can apply to caregivers too, because they must often forego cherished activities either because their loved one needs care or because the activities aren't enjoyable to go to by oneself. Tony finds it hard to enjoy weddings and the like without having me there to share the experience with him and to talk about afterward.

So envy arises easily in the life of the chronically ill and their caregivers. It can be so overpowering that it feels like it is eating us alive—and it has sometimes been like that for me. Envy is a poison, crowding out any chance at feeling peaceful and serene in the mind. In addition, the emotional stress brought on by envy exacerbates our physical symptoms. And indeed, this is not surprising since Buddhism defines an emotion as a thought plus a physical reaction to that thought.

Thankfully, mudita is a powerful antidote to the poison of envy. After becoming ill, it took me a long time to be able to easily cultivate this sublime state. At first, practicing mudita was a sheer act of will. I would learn that people I knew were going to the Mendocino coast—which used to be a favorite haunt for Tony and me—and envy would rear its ugly head. I'd remember mudita practice and try to feel joy for them, silently saying, "It's so nice they'll be seeing the ocean," but I'd be saying it through gritted teeth. It felt like fake mudita. I stuck with the practice though and slowly, slowly, slowly fake mudita started to become genuine mudita.

And this is a crucial point. Sticking with a practice even though it might feel artificial or fake still allows that practice to enter our hearts, our minds, and our bodies. This begins to change our conditioned response from a painful one (in this case, envy) to a wholesome one (in this case, joy). I continued to practice mudita even when it felt fake because when I was first taught loving-kindness practice, another one of the sublime states, I was told to stick with sending loving-kindness to ourselves and to others—even though it might not be a genuine expression of how I felt at that moment. The practice will do its work anyway, I was taught. So I persisted and cultivated fake "joy in the joy of others," hoping the feeling would become genuine. And it did.

Now when I hear about people going to a wedding or traveling or visiting family, my mind naturally moves to a feeling of joy for them. Of course, I still have an occasional "relapse" and envy again painfully arises. But because I worked on cultivating joy in the joy of others even when it didn't feel genuine, it doesn't take long for the pain of envy to subside—and even the envy itself. This has lifted a tremendous burden because few mental states rival envy as a source of self-induced suffering.

When I became house-bound and my activities were suddenly severely restricted, my initial intent in focusing on mudita was to help alleviate the suffering caused by envy. But to my surprise, after months of working with the practice, its effect turned around and the joy I felt was no longer just the joy that emanated from connecting with the joy of others, but an inward joy as if I were engaging in these cherished activities myself. So now, when Tony leaves town to visit our children and grandchildren, I not only feel joy in *his* joy of being with them, I feel as if he's there for both of us—and so I, too, am flooded with joy.

This didn't come easily though. At first when he'd call from his cell phone while he and our granddaughter Malia were off on an adventure in Los Angeles—at the Science Museum, the Santa Monica Pier, the La Brea tar pits—envy would arise in my mind and take hold of me like the tar in those pits. I *hated* not being there. I hated not being able to fulfill the dream I'd had of being an active grandparent, showing Malia all around the city of my birth. But, as has happened so many times during this illness, the Buddha's teachings came to my rescue. Again, at first, when Tony would call from one of these places and I'd hear Malia chatting or giggling in the background, cultivating mudita was a sheer act of will. I had to consciously replace envy with mudita. But now, I actually look forward to those calls. I hear the joy emanating from both of them because of their close relationship and it brings me deep and completely genuine joy.

Cultivating joy in the joy of others is a continuous challenge. As soon as I find a new interest, possibilities open up that I can't take advantage of. For example, I've become an opera buff lying in bed, but the Met is not in my future. I can't even go to the Sacramento Opera even though it's only thirty minutes away. Without mudita practice, I'd be overcome with envy. Instead, I'm happy for those who are able see opera live on the stage. And the joy I feel for them enhances my own joy when I listen to CDs or watch an opera on DVD.

The Buddha gave us a great gift when he described the cultivation of mudita. To paraphrase Shunryu Suzuki's words at the beginning of this chapter: mudita has allowed me to find perfect existence—even though my physical heath is far from perfect.

7

Soothing the Body, Mind, and Heart

*May the gentle breeze and the calm sea
protect your loved ones and friends on their journey.*
—"SOAVE SIA IL VENTO"
FROM MOZART'S *COSI FAN TUTTE*

METTA, LOVING-KINDNESS, is the act of well-wishing toward yourself and others. You settle on a set of phrases and then recite them silently, over and over. The phrases can be directed to yourself, to others as a whole, or to particular people.

These are the phrases I settled on in the early 1990s for my metta practice:

> *May I be peaceful.*
> *May I have ease of well-being*
> *May I reach the end of suffering . . .*
> *And be free.*

There's no magic to these four phrases. The cadence and meaning just work for me. "Ease of well-being" is a phrase I first heard from "metta master" Sharon Salzberg, whose book *Lovingkindness* presents one of the best descriptions of metta and the other brahma viharas. I like the phrase because it seems to direct metta at our

51

moment-to-moment experience of everyday life. It's as if I'm saying: "May I have ease of well-being as I shower . . . as I eat this
meal . . . as I lie down to nap . . . and even as I am experiencing
sickness, fatigue, and pain."

After trying out different phrases for yourself, it's best to settle
on one set. The specific content of your chosen phrases doesn't
matter so long as their theme is well-wishing. It's the act of listening to and contemplating the meaning of the phrases as you repeat
them that, over time, softens and soothes the body, mind, and
heart. In fact, now I need only silently say, "May I be peaceful"
and it sets off a relaxation response in my mind and body. They
know what's coming next! Sometimes I remove myself as the subject altogether and just lie in bed, repeating, "Peaceful, ease of
well-being, end of suffering, free."

The phrase "end of suffering" should be familiar from the first
noble truth. Recall that the Buddha said he taught two things:
dukkha and the end of dukkha. When my health didn't return, I
lay in bed, directing metta to myself. When I reached the phrase
"May I reach the end of suffering," one day I became aware that
I was wishing I'd stop feeling sick—that the physical discomfort
would *go away*, that I would *stop being sick*. Of course, wishing
for something over which I had no control only brought more
suffering. It was then that I realized that most of my suffering
came, not from the physical discomfort of the illness, but from
my mind reacting to it with thoughts like: "I don't want to be
sick"; "I hate this physical discomfort"; "What if I can never
return to work?" A shift occurred, and the end of suffering I
wished for became the end of suffering *in the mind*. In fact, I could
add "in the mind" to the end of each of my four chosen phrases,
whether I'm directing them at myself or at others. This focus on
the mind is consistent with what the Buddha meant when he
talked about the "end of dukkha."

Although I've settled on the above set of phrases for my basic metta practice, I do use other words at times. For example, while on the July 2001 retreat I wrote about earlier, I dragged myself to a talk given by Kamala Masters because, sick though I was, I loved being in her calm and serene presence. That evening, she closed her talk by directing this metta phrase to us: "Whether sick or well, may your body be a vehicle for liberation." That got my attention! I didn't replace one of my four phrases with this one, but while lying in bed, I still sometimes silently repeat: "Sick though it is, may this body be a vehicle for liberation."

Using metta phrases can also become a powerful forgiveness practice. I might repeat to myself, "Be peaceful, sweet body, working so hard to support me." When I repeat a phrase with that sentiment, I'm also forgiving myself for getting sick. It's not my body's fault that I'm sick. It's doing the best job it can to support my life.

Traditionally, metta phrases are directed at different groups of people. You start with yourself and then move progressively from those for whom it is easiest for you to evoke feelings of loving-kindness to those who are the hardest.

First, you direct the phrases at yourself. This opens your heart to the practice. It's difficult to cultivate loving-kindness for others if you're not feeling friendly toward yourself. After a time, you direct the phrases to someone for whom you feel great gratitude, who has been very generous to you. Then, you move to a person for whom you have some conflicting feelings (such as a good friend or loved one). Then, to a person you don't have an opinion about one way or another (such as your mail carrier perhaps or a checker at the supermarket). Finally, to a person whose name alone can give rise to anger, judgment, and other mind states that are a source of suffering for you.

The goal of metta practice is to cultivate loving-kindness in this fashion until it's a mental state that arises effortlessly. At that point, you'll find it increasingly natural to greet all living beings with kindness and friendliness. One of the most potent aspects of this practice is directing loving-kindness toward a person causing difficulty for you. He or she could be a family member, a doctor who doesn't take your illness seriously, or even a public figure with whom you disagree. Wishing for a person who is a thorn in your side to be peaceful and to be free from suffering may be a challenge, but it turns metta practice into a liberation practice.

During the 2008 presidential campaign, Sarah Palin became a good example of a person who bothered me who could also become an object of my loving-kindness. Some readers may react with aversion just by seeing her name on this page. (If that's not the case for you, pick another person who "lights you up" as Tony likes to say.) I've been politically active all my life and so I was involved (from my bed) in the 2008 presidential election. I didn't like Palin's political positions. I didn't like her lack of humility when asked about her reaction to being picked as a vice-presidential nominee. I soon realized that the anger I was directing at her had become such a source of stress that I was feeling it physically in my already sick body. So I did what I've done many times in the past with people to whom I'm feeling strong aversion: I went straight to my metta phrases.

First, recognizing that my reaction to her—"I don't like this about her"; "I don't like that about her"—was a great source of suffering *for me*, I began by directing metta at myself: "May I be free from the suffering that my aversion to Sarah Palin gives rise to." Then I turned to her.

"Sarah Palin: May you be peaceful. May you have ease of well-being. May you reach the end of suffering . . . and be free." As is often the case when I direct metta to difficult people in my life, just as with sympathetic joy, at first the phrases felt artificial and fake. Then I realized I'd shifted to "Sarah Palin: May you be peaceful.

May you have ease of well-being. May you reach the end of suffering . . . and be free *by seeing the error of your ways and becoming a completely different human being*." This is, of course, not exactly what the Buddha had in mind as metta practice. But as I've trained myself to do, I persisted. Soon, not only did the phrases become genuine, but I began to see in her qualities that we share. She loves her children. She wishes the best for them and hopes they'll be happy. She clings to her political views as tenaciously as I cling to mine—a shared source of suffering for us! Soon it felt like a poison had been extracted from my body, mind, and heart. Metta had been the antidote. Sarah Palin didn't get my vote, but she no longer got my rage—and I was freed from the painful negative mental state that was exacerbating my own physical symptoms.

To a sick body, a troubled mind, or a hardened heart, nothing is more soothing than metta practice. May you come to greet all of life's experiences with friendliness and loving-kindness.

8

Using Compassion to Alleviate
Your Suffering

*When the heart at last acknowledges how much pain
there is in the mind, it turns like a mother
toward a frightened child.*
—STEPHEN LEVINE, *A YEAR TO LIVE*

KARUNA, COMPASSION, is reaching out to help alleviate the suffering of ourselves and others. To do this, we must first open
our hearts to the presence of suffering in all lives. Then we can
look for ways to take compassionate action to help ease that
suffering. In this chapter, I'm going to focus on cultivating compassion for ourselves—which for many of us is harder than cultivating compassion for others.

The four sublime states are not mutually exclusive. I may call
upon more than one of them to help me through the same difficulty. Recall the story about how I cultivate mudita—joy in their
joy—when Tony and my granddaughter Malia call while they're
out and about in Los Angeles. But sometimes that call comes on a
day when I'm feeling particularly sick or blue in mood. Thanks to
mudita practice, at least I no longer feel envy when they tell me

what they're doing, but it may be too difficult for me to feel "joy in their joy."

When that happens, I turn to karuna and cultivate compassion for the suffering I'm experiencing at not being able to join them. I don't have set "compassion phrases" as I do with metta practice, so I comfort myself with whatever words come to mind, something like, "It's so hard to be at home when I want so badly to be having fun with them." Opening my heart to the suffering that arises from my desire to be with them, and then finding specific words with which I can direct compassion toward myself, always eases that suffering.

Before I became chronically ill, two teachers helped me "re-condition" my mind so that compassion became a natural response to my own suffering. The first teacher was Thich Nhat Hanh. In his book *Commentaries on the Diamond Sutra*, he describes how our body responds naturally—without thought—to its own pain:

> When our left hand is injured, our right hand takes care
> of it right away. It doesn't stop to say, "I am taking care
> of you. You are benefiting from my compassion."

Indeed, when I fell and broke my ankle, before any thoughts about it arose in my mind, my hands had already reached out to care for the pain. With practice, we can condition the mind to respond compassionately to our pain and suffering, just as our hands do. When cultivating a compassionate mental state, sometimes I look for words that address the source of the suffering, anguish, or stress. The source is, of course, what the second noble truth points to: the desire for things to be other than they are. I might silently say, "It's so hard to want so badly not to be sick." Other times, I look for words that simply open my heart to the suffering, such as, "My poor body, working so hard to feel better."

Whatever words I choose, I often stroke one arm with the hand of the other. This has brought me to tears many times, but tears of compassion are healing tears.

The second teacher who helped me learn to cultivate compassion for myself was Mary Orr who, on a Spirit Rock retreat in the late 1990s, told a story that altered my approach to life. She was describing a harried day in which she had too much to do and too little time in which to do it. (Sound familiar?) At one point, while in her car, she realized she was talking to herself in a way she would never talk to others. I don't remember her exact words, but they immediately resonated with me because of their similarity to the way I used to talk to myself:

"How stupid of me to take this route; it's always full of traffic."

"I'm so dumb, I forgot to bring my notebook."

"You clumsy idiot—you dropped your drink again."

Would I ever call Tony "dumb" or "stupid" or an "idiot"? No! And what's more, if I ever heard someone talking like this to someone I cared about—or even a stranger!—I would at least feel the impulse to intervene. Mary's story was an eye-opener for me. From then on, when I'd catch myself using that language, I'd stop and reflect on how I'd never talk to others that way. After a few months, I had "re-conditioned" my mind to treat my own difficulties with compassion.

Then I got sick and that re-conditioning unraveled.

I blamed myself for not recovering from the initial viral infection—as if not regaining my health was my fault, a failure of will, somehow, or a deficit of character. This is a common reaction for people to have toward their illness. It's not surprising, given that our culture tends to treat chronic illness as some kind of personal failure on the part of the afflicted—the bias is often implicit or unconscious, but it is nonetheless palpable. I was helped by Tony and by Spirit Rock teacher Sylvia Boorstein, who kept reminding me that this illness was just this illness and was not a personal failing on my part. In the end, it took an intense moment of physical and mental suffering for me to finally reach out to myself with compassion.

It happened on Thanksgiving. At that time, I'd been sick for a year and a half, but I was still not willing to accept that I could no longer travel to family events. So I agreed to go to Escondido where, for years, my daughter-in-law's parents, Bob and Jacqueline Lawhorn, hosted us for Thanksgiving. I planned the trip to accommodate my illness. Tony would drive down from Davis; I would get a ride to the airport and take a plane from Sacramento, which would shorten my travel time; and I'd only stay for two days.

The moment Tony picked me up at the San Diego airport and we began the forty-five-minute drive to Escondido, I knew the trip had been a mistake. We checked into our hotel and drove to the Lawhorn's house. After ten minutes of visiting, I felt so sick that the room began to spin and I couldn't focus on people. I told Jacqueline that I needed to lie down. Except for sleeping at the hotel at night, I spent that day and the next on the Lawhorn's bed. I felt no compassion for myself. I was ashamed of being sick and I blamed myself for everything my mind could come up with: undertaking the trip in the first place; taking over the Lawhorn's bedroom (which they graciously gave me, of course); not visiting with family and friends; ruining Tony's Thanksgiving. The list was long because, as Jack Kornfield likes to say, "The mind has no shame."

On Friday, Tony dropped me off at the San Diego airport. The flight was delayed two hours. I propped myself up in the chairs near the gate as best I could. I'd arranged for the Davis Airporter, a mini-van service, to pick me up at the Sacramento airport. I walked outside the terminal to find that Sacramento was socked in with tule fog—a cold, wet fog that descends on the Central Valley in winter. The van wasn't there yet, so I sat on my suitcase in the fog. Since getting sick, this was the closest I'd come to simply collapsing on the ground. When the van pulled up about fifteen minutes later, the driver told me that he had to wait for two other planes to arrive before he could drive to Davis. I got in the van and lay down on the seat to wait. It was cold and damp. Ten minutes. Fifteen minutes. Twenty minutes. My physical suffering was matched only by my mental suffering in the form of the hatred and blame I was directing at myself.

Then, suddenly, unexpectedly, there was a turning of the mind, and my heart opened. Maybe, on a subconscious level, I was recalling Mary Orr's story, and I knew I'd never treat another person the way I was treating myself. Maybe I was finally ready to receive Tony and Sylvia's compassionate reminder that this illness was not a personal failing on my part. I'm not sure what caused this change of heart and mind, but I got out of the van, explained to the driver that I was sick, and asked if he could please call the dispatcher and get permission to take me to Davis. He called, got permission immediately, and drove me home. That experience marked the beginning of my ability to treat this illness with compassion.

Immediately Make Contact

My principal compassion practice has become *tonglen*—literally "sending and taking"—from the Tibetan Buddhist tradition. We'll explore that practice in detail in chapter 11. Here, I want to write about three other practices I use to cultivate compassion for myself. I developed the first one from a generosity practice taught by Sharon Salzberg at a Spirit Rock retreat. She suggested that as soon as the thought arose to be generous in a particular way (call a friend in need, give something of ours away just because a person had admired it), we should resolve to follow through on that generous impulse even though we may subsequently try to talk ourselves out of it with thoughts like, "I'm too busy to call"; "On second thought, I want that item I was going to give away." I had used this practice for many years. Not only did it benefit others, but I found it highly amusing to reflect on the rationalizations I could come up with for talking myself out of that initial impulse to be generous: "Hmm, if I'm ever invited to the White House, I might want to wear that scarf . . ."

After that transformative experience at Thanksgiving, I looked for ways to alleviate the suffering that accompanied my illness. One day, I stumbled upon a way to change Sharon's generosity practice into a compassion practice for myself. Although the practices are quite different, I must give Sharon credit because I wouldn't have thought of mine had it not been for the wisdom of hers.

The practices are different because, instead of following through on an initial impulse to be generous, in this compassion practice I force myself to do the reverse of my initial impulse. Here's an example of how it works. If my two children haven't been in touch for a while, as soon as the thought arises, "Why don't they contact me?" I immediately contact *them*. So instead of allowing that thought, "Why don't they contact me?" to spin out into the many absurd storylines it could take ("They don't care about me"; "They'd like me better if I weren't sick"), I "cut off the mind road" (to use a Zen saying we'll learn about later) and force myself to contact them. It's as if my "penalty" for thinking that they should contact *me* is that I have to contact *them*!

The results are always uplifting and never fail to alleviate the suffering brought about by the proliferation of thoughts that simply weren't true. When I call my children, we talk about what they've been up to. We talk about my grandchildren. We share common experiences—maybe a movie on DVD or a sporting event on TV we've both seen. They may seek my advice. It always becomes clear as we're talking that they've been thinking about me. Sometimes it turns out they've been busy. (Didn't I want them to be independent as adults and to live full lives? Yes!) Sometimes it turns out they've been sick themselves.

The principal feature that Sharon's practice and my practice share is how, unless we remain vigilant by cultivating awareness—called "mindfulness" by Buddhist practitioners—the mind can talk us into or out of just about anything, no matter how counterproductive or harmful the consequences.

Here's another example of how I've used this practice. My friend Dawn tries to visit me for a short time every week. She lives two hours away but comes to Davis a few times a week for work. One time, Tony was at a meditation retreat. He'd left on a Friday. Dawn was going to visit on Tuesday. But two days after Tony left, I lost the benefit I'd been experiencing from a new treatment and had a big setback in my condition. I had to cancel our visit. She said she could visit on Wednesday instead, but I had to cancel that too. I was just too sick.

Come Friday night, I suddenly felt resentful that, knowing I wasn't doing well, Dawn hadn't checked in with me. As soon as that resentful thought arose, the "penalty" kicked in, meaning I had to cut off the negative thoughts that were about to proliferate and, instead, immediately contact her. I forced myself to pick up my laptop and send her an email. I wrote a short paragraph about my rough week and then asked how she and her family were doing. She wrote back right away. Her email started with this sentence: "I had been thinking about you, but I think I was afraid to ask you how you were doing. I won't do that again."

Here I'd been judging her negatively only to find out that, not only had she been thinking about me, but she had a reason for not getting in touch; sometimes it's just too hard for people to hear how poorly a friend is doing. In addition, it turned out she'd had a particularly busy week—hosting visitors from out of town, taking care of two of her grandchildren, negotiating the purchase of some property that was located a few hours from where she lived. A full plate indeed. Once again, the storyline I'd spun regarding someone else's motives failed to reflect what was really going on.

Practicing compassion is the act of reaching out to ourselves and to others to help alleviate suffering. By using the practice I just described, instead of allowing stressful thoughts about family and friends to proliferate and then fester, I consciously shift my mental state and take action. That action has never failed to alleviate my suffering and, as a bonus, give me a big lift.

Patient Endurance

The second way I cultivate compassion for myself is to practice *khanti*, usually translated as "patience." (Warning: it's part of another list!) Khanti is one of the ten "practices of perfection" (also called the ten *paramis*). Two of the four sublime states—metta (loving-kindness) and upekkha (equanimity)—are also on this list. The *paramis* are ten qualities that a buddha, or enlightened one, has perfected. The other seven are generosity, moral conduct, renunciation, wisdom, energy, truthfulness, and determination. In *Being Nobody, Going Nowhere*, Ayya Khema said of the perfections: "We have their seed in us. If that were not so, we would be cultivating barren ground."

Ayya Khema was a native German Jew who, after escaping the Nazis, became a Theravada Buddhist nun in Sri Lanka. She translates *khanti* as "patient endurance." At a retreat in Northern California in 1996, she told us that maintaining patient endurance is the most difficult part of Buddhist practice. Ayya Khema's rendering transforms what could be seen as a passive state of mind ("just be patient") into an active practice. Patient endurance suggests that, in addition to being patient (that is, serene and uncomplaining—two synonyms for the word "patient"), we actively "endure." The dictionary definition of *endure* includes "to survive when faced with difficulties," and "to experience hardship without giving up." I also like to compare the practice of "patient endurance" to the instruction given by Cesar Millan, the "Dog Whisperer." He tells dog owners that the most effective way to work with their pets is to maintain a "calm and assertive" mind state. In other words, take charge, but in a calm and patient manner.

I include patient endurance on my list of compassion practices because it can help alleviate our suffering as we face the many difficulties that result from being chronically ill. One recurring difficulty is the uncommon number of hours spent navigating the healthcare system, whether it's trying to get approval from an insurance company for a particular treatment or encountering a long wait or other challenge at a medical facility. Cultivating patient endurance can help caregivers too, because they often find themselves in the role of "patient advocate" for their loved one.

In general, I've found that when dealing with the healthcare system, if I don't "endure" (the assertive part of Cesar Millan's instruction), I often don't get decent service. At the same time, if I'm not "patient" (the calm part of Cesar's instruction), the frustration stemming from the interaction exacerbates my symptoms. Indeed, patience is a strong antidote to anger—a state of mind that causes so much suffering.

I've found that I need a good dose of patient endurance whenever I navigate the byzantine bureaucracy of my health insurance company. One of the most trying odysseys involved a prescription drug recommended to me by an expert in Chronic Fatigue Syndrome at Harvard. Of all things, it's produced from pig's liver. *In vitro*, it has proven to have antiviral qualities and is approved by the FDA to treat some skin conditions. To begin with, I had to get my own doctor to prescribe the drug. Not surprisingly, he was reluctant when I raised it as a possible treatment. This would be an off-label use of a drug so esoteric that it didn't even appear in his prescription drug manuals. Plus, I'd have to learn to inject myself at home. It took about a month for him to read over the research materials I provided and do his own investigation, but in the end he agreed.

With that taken care of, I could now approach my insurance company, which had no obligation to approve an off-label use of the drug. But I thought it was worth a try because the drug was so expensive. After three lengthy phone calls, I succeeded in getting approval for a three-month trial period. It was February. The representative said that the three-month trial would expire on May 15. Even though these lengthy phone calls were exhausting, I was happy with this result. Little did I know the difficulties were just beginning.

The drug is imported from New Zealand and only one pharmacy in the United States is authorized to dispense it. Even though I told them this, my insurance company insisted I use the pharmacy that it contracts with to dispense all injectable drugs. I tried over and over to explain to the representative that the pharmacy she was trying to send me to would not have access to the drug. She simply would not listen. Realizing that she was not going to budge, I wrote down the phone number for the pharmacy she said I had to call. At times during this conversation, I could feel impatience beginning to arise. I wanted to get pushy with her, but I knew it wouldn't change her position and would only exacerbate my symptoms. As it was, I was exhausted from the interaction.

"Khanti," I silently repeated to myself. "Khanti, khanti." *Patiently endure, patiently endure.*

Like a soldier on a mission she knows cannot be accomplished, I called the pharmacy she said I had to use. To my surprise, I was told, "No problem. We'll dispense it." I hung up, feeling a bit sheepish. But there was no time for reflection because I had a third call to make—to my doctor to tell him to fax the prescription to them. He did so. Mission accomplished?

Oh, no.

The next day, a woman from the pharmacy called to tell me what I already knew. I must use the pharmacy that has sole dispensing rights for the product. And she said it was *my* responsibility to call my insurance company and inform them. I felt like I was on a Moebius strip, taking action after action, but always winding up back where I started.

I took a deep breath and began again. I was already suffering from physical and mental exhaustion as a result of spending so much time on the phone. I didn't want to double the suffering by allowing impatience to take hold. So, with patient endurance as my protector, I called my insurance company and succeeded in getting the representative to phone its contracting pharmacy and get confirmation that it could not dispense the medication. A couple of phone calls later and I thought everything was in place. My doctor would re-fax the prescription to the pharmacy with the sole dispensing rights. All I had to do was wait a few hours and then call the pharmacy to arrange for shipment.

In excitement, I made the call. They were out of the drug. It had been shipped from New Zealand but was stuck in Australian customs. For the next three months, I called this pharmacy once a week. Each time, I was given a new ETA. By the time the medication arrived in the States—a year after I started researching it and three months after my doctor wrote the prescription—it was after

May 15 and the three-month trial period approved by my health insurance company had expired. Time for yet another phone call, a call in which the insurance representative told me there was no provision for an extension of an approved trial period, so I'd have to start all over if I wanted them to re-consider approving the drug. Moebius strip. Help: khanti needed!

In the end, I tried this much sought-after and hard-won medication—and it did nothing whatsoever to improve my condition. But the moral of this tale is that it might have helped (it has helped others) and so, looking back, it was the continual cultivation of patient endurance that gave me the opportunity to try the treatment. *Patience* enabled me to pursue getting the medication while keeping the exacerbation of my symptoms to a minimum. *Endurance* enabled me to make that "one more phone call" that eventually got me the result I was after.

Sometimes being sick feels like a full-time job. While I perform this work, I keep patient endurance at my side. It's a compassion practice for myself because it helps keep frustration and anger from arising—two states of mind always waiting in the wings when I have to navigate the healthcare system.

Before I learned to cultivate compassion for myself as a chronically ill person, I passively accepted whatever happened when I got to a medical facility. No matter how intense my suffering, I took no action to alleviate it—because I blamed myself for being sick. I recall, for example, an appointment I had with an ear, nose, and throat specialist in the fall of 2001 to evaluate a persistent hoarseness that was a feature of the acute phase of the illness. I dragged myself out of bed for Tony to drive us to the clinic only to find that we had to wait three hours to be seen. I tried every position I could think of to turn the waiting room chair into a reclining piece of furniture. I slumped down on my back; I slumped down on my side. Then I tried to use the chair as a bed, bending my knees to get my feet up on it and laying the middle part of my body over the hard armrest and my head on Tony's lap. The physical pain and discomfort was matched by the mental suffering that arose from blaming myself for being sick and subjecting not just me but Tony to this misery.

Six years later, I was taking an antiviral under the supervision of an infectious disease doctor. On the drive from Davis to the infectious disease clinic, I would always lay in the back of our van. But the wait at the clinic was always longer than the time it took to get there—over two hours. At the first appointment, I employed my usual techniques of first trying to turn an upright chair into a recliner and then trying to lie across Tony's lap. It took me weeks to recover from the trip. I dreaded the follow-up appointment. But at that second visit, having already begun to cultivate compassion for myself as a chronically ill person, khanti kicked in. After an hour of waiting, I calmly and politely told a staff person that I needed to lie down. To my surprise and relief, after a few minutes, she showed us to an empty room and said I could lie on the examining table until the doctor could see me. When I approached the staff person, I didn't complain, but neither was I passive. Instead, I took compassionate action on behalf of myself.

Opening Your Heart to Suffering

The third way I cultivate compassion for myself is to consciously work on opening my heart to the intense emotions—and emotional swings—that accompany chronic illness. This practice began quite unexpectedly one day in 2009 when my daughter's family had come up from Los Angeles for Labor Day weekend. I was three months into a new treatment and was feeling optimistic about its prospects. Tony and I thought this might be the one, and indeed, I'd been able to spend more time than usual visiting with everyone. But the morning after they left, I awoke feeling like my old sick self.

As I lay in bed that day, I began to fear that this treatment, like the others, was going to be a disappointment. The fear grew more and more intense, so I began to follow an instruction I learned early on in meditation practice: labeling thoughts and emotions. "Fear, fear—this is fear," I silently repeated. Sometimes it's difficult to do this work without falling prey to aversion—as in "Fear, this is fear. It's time to go away, fear. Get out of here now!" I've practiced "labeling" myriad times, both in and out of meditation, but this time something different happened. As I noted "fear . . . fear," instead of passively waiting for it to pass on through, there was a shift in consciousness and I just opened to it. Then the thought arose: "My heart is big enough to hold this fear."

And so, alongside all the other experiences of my life, I made room for fear. I felt a great spaciousness and expansiveness. Soon I became aware that a gentle smile had appeared on my lips as if to say, "Ah, yes. My old friend, fear." And so the seed was sown for a new compassion practice: opening my heart to the full range of emotions that life has in store for me.

I'd like to close our exploration of compassion with a verse from a Tibetan Buddhist master, Nyoshul Khenpo Rinpoche. Before getting sick, my mind could certainly be "exhausted" and feel as if it had been "beaten helpless," but chronic illness has the potential to exacerbate those mental states tenfold. I recite this verse as a compassion practice, to reach out to my own suffering. If you want to recite it, you can also try substituting "causes and conditions" for *karma* and "suffering-filled life" for *samsara*:

Rest in natural great peace,
this exhausted mind;
beaten helpless by karma and neurotic thought,
like the relentless fury of the pounding waves
in the infinite ocean of samsara.

9

Facing the Ups and Downs of Chronic Illness with Equanimity

Let things take their natural course.
Then your mind will become still in any surroundings,
like a clear forest pool. All kinds of wonderful,
rare animals will come to drink at the pool....
You will see many strange and wonderful things come and go,
but you will be still. This is the happiness of the Buddha.
—AJAHN CHAH

UPEKKHA, EQUANIMITY, is the fourth of the sublime states. My computer's dictionary defines equanimity as "mental calmness and evenness of temper, especially in a difficult situation." That's as good a definition as I've seen for this central Buddhist concept and practice. Dwelling in equanimity, we are able to face life's difficulties with a mind that is at peace. Indeed, some teachers equate this mental state with enlightenment—also known as awakening, liberation, or freedom.

For a chronically ill person, equanimity can be a particularly difficult state of mind to sustain—and so it helps to have both inspirational teachings and practical techniques at hand. I find the challenges fall into three categories:

- maintaining equanimity in the face of the barrage of unhelpful, inaccurate, and often insensitive comments people make about the illness
- weathering the unpredictability and uncertainty that accompanies chronic illness
- feeling overwhelmed with loss—lost health, lost job, lost friends, lost mobility, lost money

Naturally, these challenges are not entirely exclusive to those who are chronically ill. Dukkha is, after all, an equal opportunity employer. Nevertheless, chronic illness can quite often give rise to a critical need for equanimity.

Insensitive and Hurtful Comments

Anyone who is chronically ill—especially if, as in my case, the illness is not visible to others—will have encountered the first challenge many times: how are we to maintain evenness of temper and calm in the face of comments from others that, even if well-intentioned, are so off the mark that we feel misunderstood and often disregarded?

My Internet wanderings have revealed that the chronically ill are subject to remarks from family and friends that are eerily identical in content and reveal a profound ignorance about what it's like to be sick. Here's a sampling of comments, from Australia to Finland to Switzerland to my own ears in Davis:

- "But you don't look sick."
- "No wonder you're sick; you never go out."

- ▸ "I wish I had time to be sick."
- ▸ "Just drink coffee."
- ▸ "How come you can't work when you're still able to use your computer?"
- ▸ "I'm tired all the time, too."
- ▸ "I saw you pulling some weeds in your front yard; I'm glad you're healthy again."
- ▸ "If you were really that sick, you'd be in the hospital."
- ▸ "You can't be that sick if you can write a book."

Do any of those sound familiar?

Having a strong grounding in the reality of no-fixed-self, as we discussed earlier, helps one to maintain equanimity in the face of these types of comments. Ajahn Chah offers excellent advice on this point:

> If someone curses us and we have no feelings of self the incident ends with the spoken words, and we do not suffer. If unpleasant feelings arise, we should let them stop there, realizing that the feelings are not us. . . . If we do not stand up in the line of fire, we do not get shot; if there is no one to receive it, the letter is sent back.

I love that phrase: "If there is no one to receive it, the letter is sent back." This is the essence of no-fixed-self and of equanimity. With a mind that is calm and even-tempered, the insensitive comments of others are just not received. Even the word "insensitive" drops away and words are just arising and passing through our consciousness. I wish there had been "no one to receive it" when "just drink coffee" was the sole treatment offered to me by a doctor early in the chronic stage of my illness. I was devastated. It was simply too early in the illness for me to handle the comment with any semblance of equanimity. I sat there "in the line of fire"—and indeed I felt as if I'd been shot. Today I'm more likely to "not be there to receive it," in the sense that I would not take it personally. I'd know that the comment was just a reflection of his lack of skill and sensitivity as a doctor. If I felt strong enough on that day, I would "send the letter back" with some constructive feedback on the inappropriateness of the comment.

"Just drink coffee" belongs to a category of comments that caregivers have to face too: people's suggestions for treatments and cures. Countless times, Tony has told me about having to politely listen to people discourse on treatments that range from off-label use of prescription drugs to moving to a different city to the most bizarre-sounding treatments. One person told me that my body was "too acidic" and I needed to "alkalize it" by drinking baking soda and water four times a day. Two days later, another person told me my body was "too alkaline" and I needed to "acidify it" by drinking apple cider vinegar four times a day.

These comments differ from the "If you're really that sick, you'd be in the hospital" variety because the latter are insensitive and trivialize our condition. By contrast, when people offer treatments, they are genuinely trying to be helpful. Unfortunately, it's frustrating and stressful to be continually told to try things you know won't help or that you can't possibly undertake. The best way to gracefully "not be there to receive" these well-intentioned comments is to cultivate "wise speech," which we'll address in more detail later, but suffice it to say that the Buddha suggests we speak only when what we have to say is true, kind, and helpful.

Wise speech in the face of these suggestions will often be sparse speech, as in "Thanks for the suggestion." In the early 1990s, a dear friend was dying of cancer. She told me that almost every visitor arrived with a "cure" in hand, from special teas, to amulets she was to wear around her neck. Her therapist told her to say "thanks" and then promptly put the item under her bed when the person left.

Unpredictability and Uncertainty

The chronically ill face each day not knowing if we'll be able to visit with friends and family, if we can manage a trip outside of the house, if we'll have a bad reaction to a new treatment, if a doctor will be considerate or inconsiderate. We can't even predict which symptoms will hit us hard on a particular day. It's hard to stay calm and serene in these circumstances, and it's hard for caregivers too. Before I introduce two equanimity practices that I find quite helpful, I'd like to look more deeply into some of the ways that unpredictability and uncertainty show up in the lives of the chronically ill.

Activities with Others. For those of us who were always dependable when it came to keeping commitments, this sudden uncertainty in the face of people's expectations for us to make good on our plans can be a source of great anxiety and stress. Although we never feel fully healthy, the chronically ill do have days when we function better than others. We just can't predict what days those will be. As a result, we may make plans to have a friend over on a particular day, but then have to cancel that morning when we're unable to get out of bed.

Treatments. As I said, I've tried many treatments, some for symptom relief, some as possible cures. My body's response to a treatment is unpredictable. When I've undertaken one as a possible "cure," it's been a challenge to sustain a balanced state of mind that would allow me to accept success or failure with calmness and serenity. At the beginning of the experimental use of an antiviral so powerful I was monitored by three doctors, I told myself, "Maybe it will work, maybe it won't. No expectations; it's just an experiment." But when I experienced considerable improvement after six months, I thought, "This is it! Forget that 'maybe, maybe not' stuff, I'm going to get better!" Then when the positive effects of the antiviral reversed, Tony and I were crestfallen. I felt as if I'd plummeted into a deep abyss.

It was an eye-opening experience. I realized that to live gracefully with this illness, I was going to have to do a better job cultivating that evenness of temper that is at the heart of equanimity. As I write, I can think of six different major treatment regimes I've undertaken that resulted in initial success, only to be followed by disappointment. (One infectious disease doctor surmises that this might happen because my immune system adjusts to each new treatment, gradually reversing its effects.) Nothing illustrates the value of being able to ride the ups and downs of life with equanimity more than the experience of treatments that initially succeed and then fail.

Doctors. Finally, there's the unpredictability of the outcome of seeing yet another new doctor. For the chronically ill and their caregivers, the medical world is like a club we never asked to join, but now we find ourselves hanging out there all the time. When I first got sick, I approached each referral to a new specialist with high hopes, only to be let down by almost every one of them. Those with chronic illness—especially a mysterious one—have a name for this: the hot potato treatment. And I wasn't being sent from doctor to doctor because I was a difficult patient. Long before getting sick, I'd mastered the art of being a good patient: be prepared, be deferential, be succinct, don't complain too much.

I'm not indicting the medical profession. That would be painting with too broad a brush. I'm in a good position to know the harm of doing that, having spent my professional life listening to people tell nasty jokes about lawyers being worse than roadkill.

My standard in-person response was, "Good thing there were lawyers around to represent those plaintiffs in *Brown v. Board of Education*." That usually did the trick. And, naturally, I've had positive experiences with doctors. I saw an endocrinologist who was honest with me from the start. She said, "I don't know if what's wrong with you is related to your endocrine system, but I'll do my best to find out." She did indeed do her best and showed great compassion when she was unable to help me. My own primary care doctor is remarkable. He's willing to stick with me even though he can't "fix" me, he's open to my suggestions, and he gives generously of his time. He's never let me down.

That said, here's a taste of encounters with doctors that I'm sure will sound familiar to readers who inhabit the world of the chronically ill:

- A rheumatologist looked me in the eyes and told me he was going to make me well. Tony and I were so excited when we left his office. But when the tests he ordered came back normal, he coldly and bluntly told me, "Go back to your family doctor."
- A neurologist told me at my first appointment that I would be his patient. He regaled Tony and me with his expertise about post-viral syndromes, talking at length about the immune and the nervous systems. As we did with the rheumatologist, we left his office exhilarated, given his optimism about what he could do for me. But when we returned for a follow-up appointment, he showed a cursory interest in me, focusing instead on impressing the medical student he had in tow. I was treated as tangential to whatever agenda he had in mind with this student. He spent about ten minutes with us and was gone, offering no help. Tony and I left feeling utterly

deflated. I still can't explain why the follow-up visit bore no resemblance to the initial work-up.

- An infectious disease doctor asked me to email him ahead of our appointment the results of my own research into possible treatments. I spent hours researching online, writing, and then editing an email for him that would be succinct but thorough—at some cost to my health and well-being. When he came into the examining room, he acknowledged having received the email but said he hadn't read it. When I politely expressed disappointment, he was miffed and said he'd call me when he'd read it. I never heard from him.

- Another infectious disease doctor asked me to make a graph of my day-to-day progress on the antiviral treatment he was monitoring. I painstakingly created a chart based on notes I kept in a daily journal. When I was responding well to the medication, he loved my chart, even calling colleagues into the room to look at it. But when the medication's benefits began to wear off, he wouldn't even look at the chart I had so carefully updated since my last appointment. Even worse, he blamed me for the failure of the antiviral. I wasn't resting enough. I wasn't doing the right kind of exercise. I rested at every opportunity, and exercise? It was an exercise just getting to the appointment. When it was clear his treatment wasn't going to work for me, he dropped me . . . like a hot potato.

Equanimity Practices

In the 1990s, when the Thai Forest monk Ajahn Jumnian came for his annual visit to Spirit Rock, I faithfully attended. Bubbling over—as he always was—with joy and laughter, one day he suddenly began discoursing on equanimity. I got out a pen and took these notes:

> When people say, "Ajahn, let's go for a beautiful walk," fine I'll go. If they don't ask, that's fine too. I don't expect a walk to be any more satisfying than sitting alone. It could be hot or windy out there. If people bring me delicious food, great. If they don't, great. I need to diet anyway. If I'm feeling good, that's okay. If I'm sick, that's okay too. It's a great excuse to lie down.

These few sentences, scribbled on a scrap of paper as Jack Kornfield translated, have become the centerpiece of equanimity practice for me. I rediscovered the notes several years after becoming sick. Reading them with my new circumstance in mind, I understood that the essence of equanimity is accepting life as it comes to us without blaming anything or anyone—including ourselves. I'd been getting despondent when a treatment didn't work and becoming angry when a doctor didn't live up to my expectations. I was trying to control the uncontrollable. Some treatments work. Some don't. Some doctors come through for us. Some don't.

The challenge is to not let this insight slip into indifference, because indifference is a subtle aversion to life as it comes to us. Indifference turns the serene acceptance of "Things are as they are" into "Things are as they are—so who cares?" This is why my notes from Ajahn Jumnian's visit and my memory of the joy that emanated from him are still so inspiring. Now I cultivate equanimity by saying, "If this medication helps, that will be great. If it doesn't, no blame. It wasn't what my body needed." "If this doctor turns out to be responsive, that will be nice. If he or she doesn't, that's okay. Any given doctor is going to be how he or she is going to be. It's not in my control."

I try to remember Ajahn Jumnian's little gem when I'm faced with the unpredictability of being able to participate in activities or visit with people. Early on in my illness, I bought tickets to the Sacramento Opera's production of *Carmen*. I thought that even if Tony and I could only stay for Act I of the matinee, it would still be a wonderful experience. But on the day of opera, I was too sick to leave the house. I was terribly resentful and angry that we couldn't go through with the plans I'd so carefully made—including calling to find out how long each act lasted and where the closest disabled parking was. The resentment and anger turned to tears, making it harder for Tony. I simply did not have a strong enough equanimity practice to handle the uncertainty and unpredictability that had so unexpectedly become my constant companion in life.

Fast-forward six years. An old family friend was in town and Tony invited him to dinner. I carefully arranged my week so I wouldn't have other commitments in the days leading up to the dinner. This greatly increased the likelihood that I'd be able to join him and Tony for a bit even though I rarely leave the bedroom after 5:30. But on the evening he came, I was too sick to visit. Had we happened to have scheduled the dinner the night before, I would have been able to socialize for a while.

However, I didn't react the same way I had to the missed opera experience. I didn't lie in the bedroom and cry that night. Instead I recalled Ajahn Jumnian's words and said to myself, "If I could have joined them, that would have been nice. Since I can't, that will be okay too. I'll lie in bed and listen to music or find a movie on TV."

A second equanimity practice comes from another Thai Forest monk, Ajahn Chah, whom we've heard from before. In his book

A Still Forest Pool, he offers a statement so powerful that I'd c‌mitted it to memory long before getting sick:

> If you let go a little, you will have a little peace. If you let go a lot, you will have a lot of peace. If you let go completely, you will know complete peace and freedom. Your struggles with the world will have come to an end.

I love this teaching because it allows me to take baby-steps in the direction of equanimity. I've found that before I can even take that first step and "let go a little," I first have to recognize the suffering that arises from my desire for certainty and predictability. Just seeing the suffering in that desire loosens its hold on me, whether it's wanting so badly to be at a family gathering or clinging to the hope for positive results from a medication or desiring for a doctor not to disappoint me. Once I see the dukkha in the mind, I can begin to let go a little. As soon as I do that, I get a taste of freedom that motivates me to let go a little more.

I used this practice while waiting for my ankle to be x-rayed. There I was, twenty-four hours after slipping down the two steps, my ankle still throbbing in pain, my knees bruised from crawling around the house, my body aching in fatigue from sitting in a wheelchair way beyond my capacity to be in an upright position. As thoughts whirled around about whether I could handle this injury on top on my illness, I searched for help in coping with the dukkha in my body and in my mind. Help came from Ajahn Chah's teaching on letting go. I thought, "I'm suffering because I don't want this to be happening but, like it or not, it *is* happening, so can I let go just a little—just a baby-step?" I could. And, having done that, I could take another baby step. After a few minutes, I was flooded with equanimity—with the taste of freedom that comes with peaceful acceptance of the unexpected complications that arise in our lives.

Our tendency is, of course, to want our desires to be fulfilled. But if our happiness depends on that, we've set ourselves up for a life of suffering. The strength of our equanimity in the face of not having our desires fulfilled is the measure of whether we will know the peace and freedom to which Ajahn Chah refers. It's the measure of whether, as he said, our "struggles with the world will have come to an end."

Imagine living in a world where we've let go completely and it's okay if we can't go to that family event, it's okay if a medication doesn't help, it's okay if a doctor is disappointing. Just imagining it inspires me to let go a little. Then it's easier to let go a lot. And every once in a while, I let go completely and, momentarily, bask in the glow of that blessed state of freedom and serenity that is equanimity.

Loss

Facing losses that feel overwhelming—from lost health to lost friends to lost livelihood—deeply challenges our cultivation of equanimity. But we can sometimes find teachings and practices in the most unexpected of places. One day I was watching an interview on television with the actress Susan Saint James. Three weeks before the interview, her fourteen-year-old son, Teddy, was killed in a plane crash. Her husband and another son were seriously injured and several of the crewmembers died. In the interview, Saint James talked about how close she was to Teddy because he was her youngest child and the only one still living at home. In addition, due to his work as head of NBC sports, her husband, Dick Ebersol, was gone much of the time. She said that she and Teddy were like roommates and had become best friends.

Then, emanating deep calm and acceptance, she made this most astonishing comment: "His was a life that lasted fourteen years." I gasped. Could I make that statement with such equanimity should one of my children or grandchildren die? I still don't know the answer to that question. But Susan Saint James's words and the serenity with which she spoke them entered my heart that day. Ever since, when I find myself in grief and despair over the many losses I've had to face due to my illness, her words are my equanimity practice.

When I feel myself mourning my lost career as a law professor or a lost friendship, I say to myself, "This was a career that lasted twenty years"; or "This was a friendship that lasted twenty-five years." If I feel overwhelmed by the loss of my health and its consequences, I say to myself, "This was a body that was illness-free long enough to be active in raising my children and to not be a burden to them when they were young; to be a part of their weddings; to teach and be of personal support to many law students; to travel and keep company with Tony out in the world."

Inspired by Susan Saint James's courage, which reinforces the teachings of the Buddha that I've learned, I'm able to say these equanimity phrases without bitterness. I can even be genuinely grateful for those years. When overcome with the losses you've encountered, be you chronically ill or the caregiver for a loved-one who is chronically ill, I encourage you to try the equanimity practice I cobbled together from the words of a remarkable woman facing the most devastating loss we can imagine.

Turnarounds and Transformations

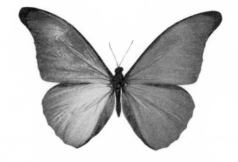

10

Getting Off the Wheel of Suffering

Nothing whatsoever should be clung to.

—BUDDHADASA BHIKKHU

MANY TEACHERS suggest starting Buddhist practice by learning how to meditate, but because of my academic background, I was compelled to hit the books first and do some research. Such was my need to put scholarship first, that soon after becoming interested in Buddhism in 1992, I researched and wrote a twenty-page paper, complete with footnotes that referenced over three dozen books. I titled it "Introduction to Buddhism." Given that I can't recall giving this little piece of scholarship to anyone, I appear to have been introducing Buddhism to myself.

While engaging in this scholarly study, I adopted a strategy that served me well: if I came upon a teaching that I didn't understand, I skipped it. That was my first relationship to the wheel of suffering. I skipped it and moved to a teaching that was more accessible.

I started my study with a book we already owned: *What the Buddha Taught*, written in 1959 by the Sri Lankan monk and scholar Walpola Rahula. In 1992, when I took it off the bookshelf, his work was still considered by many the seminal guide for introducing Westerners to Buddhism. It was not an easy read, especially in contrast to the dozens of user-friendly books on Buddhism now available. When I reached Rahula's discussion of the doctrine called *paticca-samuppada*—the "wheel of suffering" or, as it's more commonly known, "dependent origination"—I very well might have been derailed in this new spiritual pursuit had I not just skipped over it. His use of phrases such as "conditioned genesis" and "cessation of volitional formations" had my mind spinning.

But years later, my meditation practice well-established, I tackled that teaching again through the writings of Ayya Khema and S.N. Goenka and it began to make sense. In particular, I learned a lot from *When the Iron Eagle Flies* by Ayya Khema and *Vipassana Meditation as Taught by S.N. Goenka* by William Hart.

Paticca-samuppada can be translated in many different ways. While the most common translation is "dependent origination," I've chosen "the wheel of suffering" because it's so descriptive of our experience. With the caveat that this will not be a comprehensive nor scholarly analysis, I'm going to jump on in the middle of the twelve steps on this wheel or chain of suffering and explain how I use these teachings as a practical tool to help alleviate the mental suffering that accompanies chronic illness.

As we go through life, we repeatedly encounter mental and physical contacts through our six senses. (Buddhism, like other Indian philosophical systems, includes the mental faculty that coordinates our perceptions as a sixth sense.) We experience these contacts as pleasant, unpleasant, or (less frequently) as neutral sensations. If the experience of the contact is *pleasant*, we want more of it, which is desire. If the experience of the contact is *unpleasant*, we want it to go away, which is simply another form of desire—the desire for it to go away—usually referred to in Buddhism as aversion. The Pali term for this desire/aversion, as we discussed above, is *tanha*. I like to refer to *tanha* as "want/don't want"—since it pretty well describes one of the two mental states I'm in a good part of each day!

The mind then latches on to this desire or aversion, sticking to it like glue. This part of the process is varyingly referred to as clinging, grasping, or attachment. Once we've latched on to desire or aversion like this, there's no turning back. This latching on gives rise to a sense of a solid self—as if the glue has dried. In short, we are reborn moment to moment into self-identities we create by clinging or attaching to our desires and aversions.

We then have to live out the consequences of the birth—or re-birth, if you like—we have taken each moment. Those consequences are what's meant by *karma*, and living out those consequences is the ripening or fruition of karma.

Take a simple example. There's a contact with the world in the form of someone merging in front of us in traffic even though we have the right-of-way. Note that the contact involves more than one sense: the eyes see the car merge, the ears hear the car move, the sixth sense thinks, "He's cutting in front of me even though I have the right-of-way." The part of the contact involving the mind is experienced as an unpleasant sensation. Before we can stop ourselves, we react with aversion to the unpleasantness. In fact, we can't shake the aversion. It takes hold of us, sticking like glue, and we're right on course for "becoming" and being "reborn" that very moment as a cranky person. And there you have it: suffering—the first noble truth.

The good news is that we can break the cycle before we get to that place of suffering by becoming mindful right at that moment *before* an unpleasant sensation gives rise to the desire that things be other than they are. S.N. Goenka refers to this as "learning to observe [unpleasant sensations] objectively." He says that between he contact and the reaction to it—the desire or aversion—stands a crucial step: "When we learn to observe sensation without reacting in craving and aversion, the cause of suffering does not arise and suffering ceases."

That split-second between the experience of a pleasant or unpleasant sensation and the arising of desire for the former or aversion to the latter is the doorway out, our opportunity to get off the wheel of suffering. We can't avoid the arising of sensation or feeling after a contact—touching a hot stove is going to feel unpleasant! But Ayya Khema says that the practice is to see that sensation as just a sensation without owning it. After all, she says, if we really "owned" our sensations in the sense of being fully able to control them, we'd never let our sensations and feelings be anything but pleasant! And this is also what S.N. Goenka means when he says we should learn to observe sensations objectively.

When someone merges in front of us in traffic even though we have the right-of-way, we can just observe that the sensation is unpleasant and leave the experience at that—without reacting to it as anything more than one of the thousands of momentary contacts we encounter every day. Not only will we see the truth of impermanence, but suffering will not arise and, before we know it, we've moved on to the next contact of the day, which might just be a sympathetic smile from another driver.

This takes us to a practice I developed that combines the teachings of the wheel of suffering with the four sublime states—even though they may appear to be an unlikely partnership.

Practicing with the Wheel of Suffering and the Four Sublime States

The idea for this practice began with a teaching from the wise and wonderful Sylvia Boorstein, whom I mentioned above. Sylvia is one of Spirit Rock's founding teachers. In her book *Happiness Is an Inside Job* she tells the story of how she and her husband, Seymour, were visiting a ski resort in Europe. As Sylvia watched people learning to ski, she recalled all the times she and Seymour had tackled the slopes together before reaching the age where it would no longer be safe for them to do so. Just as her mind began to "wobble" as she calls it (my wobble would have been straight to the unpleasant mental feeling of envy), she looked around at all the fun people were having and suddenly felt great delight in their joy, especially that of a little girl who was just learning to ski. And so, with her wisdom mind, Sylvia turned that approaching negative mind state into the sublime state of joy in the joy of others.

Shortly after I read this chapter in Sylvia's book, Tony and I were talking about how we seem to be hard-wired to experience contact as pleasant, unpleasant, or neutral. This includes both physical and mental contact: I can no more turn touching a hot stove into a pleasant experience than I can turn hearing a racist comment into one. The question for me becomes whether I can get off the wheel of suffering at that point, before the unpleasant experience of something like a racist comment turns into aversion—the "don't want" side of desire. Once I react with aversion, clinging isn't far behind and before I know it I've completed the cycle and have been "reborn" as person so full of anger that I'm unable to take wise action to counter the comment.

I had been mulling over both Sylvia's skiing chapter and this discussion with Tony when the time came for me to try to nap. I lay in bed, my body aching with flu-like symptoms, my heart pounding with wired fatigue. Of course, I was experiencing this as an unpleasant physical sensation. My mind began its usual movement—Sylvia's "wobble"—from the experience of the unpleasant sensation to aversion to that sensation, when I realized how to find that doorway out that S.N. Goenka and others talk about. In other words, I found a way to break the vicious cycle of suffering. I did it by consciously moving my mind toward one of the four sublime states.

As I lay in bed, the flu-like symptoms were indeed physically unpleasant. But, instead of mindlessly allowing aversion to arise as I had done thousands of times in the past, I realized I had a choice of where to put my mind. So I consciously moved my mind to loving-kindness, silently repeating, "Dear sweet, innocent body, working so hard to support me." Directing this well-wishing at my own body was my doorway out of dukkha. I got off the wheel of suffering. I was free from aversion to my illness and from all that can follow from that aversion—for example, becoming and being reborn as a bitter and resentful person.

Of course, I was so conditioned to moving right into aversion or desire that this breakthrough didn't mean I no longer had to work at all this. Every day, I have to work on learning to observe sensations objectively and sometimes I don't make it out that door. But I practice hard at it.

I practice by, first, becoming mindful that, yes, this bodily sickness feels unpleasant. Then I consciously move my mind to whatever sublime state works for me at that moment. So I may move to loving-kindness as described above. Or I may move to compassion, silently saying, "It's so hard to feel this sick. It's hard to feel under attack by some mystery virus and not be able to find a treatment that works." Often as I say this, I pet one arm with the hand of my other arm—a practice I learned from Thich Nhat Hanh in his *Commentaries on the Diamond Sutra*. Sometimes my mind inclines toward equanimity and I silently say, "This is how it is. My body is sick. It's okay. This is just how it is." Recently, I've developed the ability to cultivate joy in the joy of others so that, as I lay in bed experiencing the unpleasant bodily sensations that accompany the illness, I feel happy for those who are in good health.

I also use joy in the joy of others in the same way Sylvia did.

When I'm not able to visit with my family in the front of the house and I experience it as an unpleasant mental sensation or feeling, instead of moving to aversion and all the suffering that inevitably follows, I consciously move my mind to mudita, feeling joy that they are able to spend this time with each other.

I have used this practice of combining awareness of the wheel of suffering with the four sublime states to help me through the most difficult of circumstances. For example, I had a period of two days and nights when I stopped sleeping. It wasn't insomnia. The flu-like malaise and the oppressive, heart-pounding fatigue were just too strong to allow my body to fall asleep, just as someone in pain can't sleep. When people who are well have a couple of sleepless nights, they don't feel good during the day, but they can function. I'm only slightly restored when I have a good night's sleep, so you can imagine how not sleeping at all affected me.

During those two sleepless nights, my previous reaction would have been to go straight from the unpleasant physical sensation to aversion followed by misery. I would have lain in bed getting increasingly frustrated and angry at my body. Instead, I consciously moved my mind among the sublime states.

At 2:00 A.M., I'd be invoking loving-kindness: "Sweet body, trying so hard to sleep."

At 3:00 A.M., compassion: "It's so hard to lie in bed, needing to sleep but not being able to."

At 4:00 A.M., equanimity: "This is how things are; my body is not able to sleep right now."

On the third night, I slept.

I'm convinced that using these practices to keep the unpleasant sensations from turning to aversion kept my symptoms from increasing more than they already had, and eventually allowed the flare-up to subside. I'm so grateful that these two Buddhist practices teamed up to help me through that difficult time.

II

Tonglen: Spinning Straw into Gold

O that my monk's robe
were wide enough
to gather up all
the suffering people
in this floating world.

—RYOKAN

TONGLEN IS A COMPASSION PRACTICE from the Tibetan Buddhist tradition. Nonetheless, I find that Ryokan's Zen poem above captures for me the essence of tonglen. Of course, they are both inspired by the example of the Buddha.

When I first got sick, it didn't take long for me to accumulate a collection of healing CDs from a variety of spiritual traditions. They had one thing in common: I was instructed to breathe *in* peaceful and healing thoughts and images, and to breathe *out* my mental and physical suffering. In tonglen practice, however, the instruction is to do just the opposite. We breathe *in* the suffering of the world and breathe *out* whatever kindness, serenity, and compassion we have to give. It's a counter-intuitive practice, which is why the Buddhist nun and teacher Pema Chödrön says that tonglen reverses ego's logic.

Tonglen practice was brought to Tibet from India in the eleventh century as part of a group of teachings known as the "seven points of mind training," a collection of fifty-nine "slogans" for practicing the path of compassion. The practice of tonglen is described in the slogan: Train in taking and sending alternately; put them on the breath.

Those two phrases don't give us a lot of guidance, but for hundreds of years this slogan, along with the other fifty-eight, has been a favorite subject for commentary by Tibetan masters. Recent commentaries can be found in the writings of Chögyam Trungpa, Dilgo Khyentse, and Pema Chödrön, among others. These commentaries flesh out the meaning of each slogan. And so tonglen becomes: Breathe in the suffering of others; breathe out kindness, serenity, and compassion. We are, in effect, breathing out the sublime states of mind introduced above.

I had learned tonglen practice before getting sick, but I didn't use it very often. Now it's my principal compassion practice. My bond with tonglen occurred on the first day I returned to work, six months after getting sick in Paris.

Like everyone else around me, I couldn't believe I wasn't well enough to continue with my profession, at least on a part-time basis. So a half-hour before my scheduled class, Tony dropped me off at the front door of the law school. It was the second week of January 2002. I took the elevator up one floor to my office. I was to teach Marital Property to second- and third-year students. As soon as I sat down in my office chair, I knew I was too sick to be there. I began to panic, so I lay down on a couch in the office. Unexpectedly, my thoughts turned to the millions of people who must go to work every day even though they're sick. I realized that many of these people were in a worse position than I was—if they didn't go to work, they wouldn't be able to pay the rent or buy food for their families.

I'd been in the work force for dozens of years but had never before thought about people being forced to work while sick. As I was contemplating this, I began to breathe in their suffering (which, as a sick person myself, now included my own suffering). Then I breathed out what kindness, serenity, and compassion I had to give. To my surprise, the panic subsided and was replaced with a feeling of deep connection to all these people. Even more astonishing was the realization that, as sick as I was at that moment and as preoccupied as I was about the task awaiting me in less than ten minutes, there was still some kindness, serenity, and compassion inside me to send to others on the out-breath.

A few minutes later, I arose from the couch, took a chair with me, and, for the first time in twenty years, taught a class while sitting down. For the next two and a half years of part-time teaching, I used tonglen in my office, followed by adrenaline in the classroom to get me through the work week. Only Tony saw the devastating effect that continuing to work had on me as I went straight from the car to the bed and stayed there until the next class I had to teach. When I think of those years, tonglen and that couch in my office are inseparable in my mind. I don't know how I would have survived without both.

After that first day back at work, I began to use tonglen all the time. I'd use it while waiting for the results of medical tests. It took me out of my small world—out of exclusive focus on my illness—and connected me with all the people caught up in the medical system who were anxiously waiting to hear the results of tests. It never failed to amaze me that no matter how worried I was, there was always some serenity, some good wishes, some compassion inside me to send out to others in the same situation. Finding our own storehouse of compassion is the wonder of tonglen practice.

Gradually, the fear over my test results would diminish, and I could wait with equanimity to see what the world had in store for me next.

I love that tonglen is a two-for-one compassion practice. The formal instruction is to breathe in the suffering of others and breathe out kindness, serenity, and compassion. But the effect of repeated practice is that we connect with our own suffering, anguish, stress, discomfort. So as we breathe in the suffering of others concerning a struggle we share with them, we are breathing in our own suffering over that struggle as well. As we breathe out whatever measure of kindness, serenity, and compassion we have to give, we are offering those sublime states to ourselves too. *All* beings are included.

Yet there came a day when I reached my limit with tonglen. I tried the practice on Thanksgiving Day, two and a half years after I got sick, while lying in my bedroom and listening to the sound of my family chatting and laughing in the front of the house. I tried breathing in the sadness and sorrow of all the people who were in the same house as their family on Thanksgiving, but were too sick to join in the festivities. It was too much. I just couldn't hold everyone's suffering without crying. So I cried.

But four years later, in a similar circumstance, the practice worked. It was a measure of how tonglen had slowly worked its magic. My second grandchild, Camden Bodhi, was born in September 2007. I hosted a welcoming party for her that, as it turned out, I could not attend. When I set the plan in motion in the spring, I was halfway through a year-long experimental antiviral treatment that appeared to be working. But six months later, on the day of the party, I was too sick to take the hour-long trip to Berkeley. I lay in bed that day, thinking about friends and family who had gathered to celebrate my granddaughter's birth and I was overcome with sorrow.

First, I tried mudita practice—cultivating joy in the joy of those who were at the celebration. It helped, but I continued to feel sad and disheartened by my inability to attend, by thoughts about the good time I was missing, by the feeling that I had let others down. So I turned to tonglen. I breathed in the suffering of all those who were unable to be with their families on a special day of celebration. As I did this, I was aware I was breathing in my own sadness and sorrow, but, unlike that Thanksgiving Day, I was able to hold the suffering—to care for it—without feeling overcome by it. I then breathed out kindness, serenity, and compassion for them and for myself. The connection I felt with all those people was powerful and moving.

If you feel hesitant to try tonglen for fear that breathing in other people's suffering could overwhelm you, you're not alone. Here's the response given by the eco-philosopher and Buddhist scholar Joanna Macy when that very concern was raised at a Spirit Rock workshop. First, she reassured the woman asking the question that her capacity to hold others' suffering was greater than she imagined. Then she said:

If you really could alleviate all the suffering in the world by breathing it in, wouldn't you?

Of course, this is a hypothetical and so not a realistic assessment of the effect of practicing tonglen. Indeed at times we may cry in response to breathing in the suffering in the world, but it's compassionate crying—a perfectly appropriate response. And those moments when we *can* hold the suffering of the world on the in-breath and breathe out whatever kindness, serenity, and compassion we have to give are like turning straw into gold.

12

With Our Thoughts We Make the World
AN APPRECIATION OF BYRON KATIE

*In our everyday life,
our thinking is 99% self-centered.
"Why do I have suffering? Why do I have trouble?"*
—SHUNRYU SUZUKI

SEVERAL YEARS BEFORE I GOT SICK, I attended a retreat in Northern California led by Ayya Khema. In it, she gave a talk on the nature of thought. According to my notes, she said at one point: "Thoughts are just there, like the air around us. They arise but are arbitrary and not reliable. Most of them are just rubbish, but we believe them anyway."

I took her words to heart and, before getting sick, had become quite adept at applying this teaching. Especially while in formal meditation, I could watch a thought arise in the mind, treat it as impersonal energy, and let it pass through. I knew I couldn't control the content of thoughts that arose, but I also knew it wasn't the content that led to suffering. Suffering arose when I "believed" the thought, when I believed its content was a valid reflection of reality. I knew, for example, that the thought "My Torts class won't go well today" didn't mean that the class wouldn't be just fine. "Believing a thought" is another way of saying that we're clinging to it, continuing to go round and round on the wheel of suffering.

By the time the Parisian Flu hit, I had a good understanding of the nature of thoughts and the circumstances under which they gave rise to suffering. But put me in the sick bed all day and suddenly my thoughts seemed anything but impersonal. As for Ayya Khema's statement that thoughts are arbitrary and not reliable, I now believed every one of them held the force of Absolute Truth:

"I'll never feel joy again."

"No doctor wants to treat me."

"All my friends have abandoned me."

"I've ruined Tony's life."

Thoughts and suffering were now marching hand in hand in my life.

As I often do when I'm overwhelmed by dukkha, I turned to the Buddha for help. One of the most famous lines from a small book called the *Dhammapada* came to mind: "With our thoughts we make the world."

With my thoughts, I had made a world of suffering to live in. And the thoughts had a stranglehold on me because I believed they were true—that I *was* ruining Tony's life, that I *wouldn't* feel joy again. In confronting the suffering that my thoughts were causing, I was helped by an inspiring teacher named Byron Katie. Katie, as everyone calls her, encourages us to question the validity of what she refers to as our stressful thoughts. I highly recommend her books and her website. Using what she calls "The Work" or inquiry, she sets forth a five-step method for revealing the suffering that follows when we believe our thoughts. Along with the Buddha's teachings, Byron Katie's inquiry is the most powerful tool I've found to help with the challenges of being chronically ill.

When I became house-bound, it wasn't long before I started to worry about the fate of my friendships. But instead of examining the possible reasons why friends might not be visiting, I kept thinking over and over, "My friends should not stop coming to see me." Each time the thought arose, it was accompanied by hurt and anger. This one thought became an ever-present source of suffering in my life.

Inquiry Practice

Byron Katie shows us how to question the validity of thoughts that are a source of stress or suffering.

In the first step, we ask whether the thought is true, and in this case I answered, "Yes, it is true that my friends should not stop coming to see me."

In the second step, we ask whether we can absolutely know that it is true. On this, I was not as certain: "Do I *absolutely* know it's true? Hmm. Maybe this requires a bit more investigation . . ."

The third step in questioning the validity of a stressful thought is to notice how we react when we believe the thought. When I believed the thought, "My friends should not stop coming to see me," I reacted with anger and I felt hurt, almost as if I were being wounded physically.

The fourth step is to reflect on who we'd be without the thought. I closed my eyes and imagined who I'd be . . . and my answer was: "I'd be living this day as it unfolds—seeing what it has to bring, instead of just being focused on who may or may not visit." Without the stressful thought, "My friends should not stop coming to see me," I felt liberated, as if a heavy burden had been lifted—the burden of constantly worrying about the state of my friendships.

Then comes the counter-intuitive *fifth step*, when Katie asks us to come up with a "turnaround." A turnaround is a statement of the stressful thought in a way that's opposite from its original expression. So I tried saying, "My friends *should* stop coming to see me."

On first read, that sounds absurd, but when I turned the original thought around this way, I saw that there were genuine reasons why my friends might not be visiting. Many people are uncomfortable around others who are sick—they may be afraid they'll get sick or perhaps seeing someone who is sick reminds them of their own mortality. They might not be visiting because they think it will be too hard on me. Maybe they feel bad about sharing all the enjoyable activities they're involved in since I'm stuck at home. In addition, people get caught up in the busyness of their lives; they often barely have time to spend with their own families. Perhaps they're having medical problems themselves; how would I know since I'm no longer in contact with them?

Working on the turnaround led to two other unexpected insights. First, while generating all these possible reasons why friends might not be visiting, it dawned on me for the first time that just because they weren't visiting—or even calling me—didn't mean they weren't thinking kind thoughts about me and hoping that I'd get better. Over the years, hadn't there been people I could have contacted when they were sick but didn't? Absolutely.

Second, I realized that the reasons friends weren't coming to see me had to do with what was going on in their minds, not mine. I can't control the thoughts that arise in my *own* mind. How could I imagine I could control what my friends were thinking? No wonder when, in the fourth step, I reflected on who I'd be without the stressful thought, I felt as if a heavy burden had been lifted. As the Buddha said, with our thoughts we make our world. I had created a bitter and resentful world.

Working with Byron Katie's inquiry showed me that I had spun so many emotionally packed tales about why friends weren't visiting that I hadn't stopped to examine what the true reasons might be. It wasn't my friends who were the source of my suffering; it was my own unexamined thinking about them. That wound I was feeling turned out to be self-inflicted. Now it could begin to heal. I stopped blaming friends for not visiting and I no longer assumed they didn't care about me.

I use Byron Katie's inquiry all the time. I even used it when I was stuck-like-glue on a stressful thought about her! Tony was planning to attend a daylong session with her at Spirit Rock. I really wanted to go. I felt like I knew her personally from her books and from videos posted on her website, where I could watch her in one-on-one dialogues with people in which she guides them through the "four questions and a turnaround."

So, as Katie would have suggested, I wrote down the thought that was causing me so much stress: "I really want to go to Spirit Rock on Saturday to see Katie." Then, I subjected the thought to her five-step process. Not only was it true that I wanted to go, but, unlike my example with friends not visiting, this time I thought it was "absolutely true." Katie says that starting with these two questions—Is the thought true? and Can we absolutely know it's true?—forces us to commit one way or the other. Then we can watch how the mind acts to defend our response. "Don't tell me I might not want to go to Spirit Rock. I absolutely do!"

Then I moved to the third question and asked how I reacted when I believed the thought "I really want to go to Spirit Rock on Saturday to see Katie." I reacted with anger and resentment. I felt like a victim in an unfair world. But when I moved to the fourth question and asked who I'd be without the thought, I immediately saw that I'd be a person living in the present moment, which happened to be a beautifully sunbathed Tuesday—days away from the Saturday event.

Working through these four questions was helpful, but, as can happen, the stressful thought persisted until I got to the magical turnaround. I turned the thought around to "I don't want to see Katie on Saturday." Then, following Katie's instructions, I looked for at least three genuine reasons why the turnaround might be true. I actually came up with five. First, it would take me a week, maybe several, to recover from the trip. Second, the event was going to be very crowded so I might not be able to find a comfortable place to sit or lie down. Third, I might catch a cold or the flu from someone who was there. Fourth, by seeing Katie in person I might not improve my inquiry skills any more than I would by continuing to watch her videos on my computer. Fifth, she could be a big disappointment! (I know from watching her in dialogue with others on video that Katie would have loved that last turnaround.)

After putting all this down on paper—as she suggests we do because of the power of the written word—I was fully content not to go on Saturday. I had let go of the stressful thought and it never returned, even as I saw Tony off to see her.

One day, I wrote down a thought that, understandably, was a great source of suffering:

"I hate being sick."

It was true, and I felt it was *absolutely* true. But how did I react when I believed the thought? Bitter, frustrated, singled-out by the world. Who would I be without the thought? I'd be a woman, lying on a comfortable bed in a quiet room, enjoying the exquisite play of sunlight on the tail of the squirrel who was visible outside my window. Katie says she isn't telling us to give up the stressful thought but to drop it just long enough to see who we'd be without it.

Then I turned the thought around:

"I love being sick."

Could I possibly come up with three genuine reasons why thi turnaround might be true? I thought not, but I let ink from my pen flow onto the page anyway. When I was finished, I'd come up with twelve reasons. Here's what I wrote, unedited, and in the order I wrote it:

- I don't answer to an alarm clock.
- I have the perfect excuse to avoid events and people I don't want to be with.
- I have lots of time to be with Tony and Rusty, our dog.
- I'm getting to know Bridgett, my daughter-in-law, really well for the first time in over a dozen years.
- My life is pretty quiet and peaceful.
- I'm never stuck in traffic.
- I don't have to work.
- There's nothing I have to read or study.
- My "To Do" list is very short.
- Most of my day is unplanned, so in summer, I can lie down in the backyard before it gets too hot and in winter, wait until it warms up to do so.
- I've met some people I wouldn't have otherwise known.
- Being home sick allowed Winnie, our previous dog, to live another year since, in that last year, she couldn't be home alone.

I can't say that since performing this inquiry, I haven't again believed the thought "I hate being sick" and suffered as a consequence. I have dozens of times—this work is not necessarily about ridding oneself of stressful thoughts but rather about examining their validity. But the work I did that day on "I hate being sick" is right there, on paper, and re-reading it is always helpful.

Then came the day when I tackled this stressful thought:

"I am sick."

I was surprised at the number of genuine reasons why the turn-around was true:

"I am not sick."

My mind isn't sick—I'm able to do this inquiry. My heart isn't sick—I can express love and be of help to others. Not all of my body is sick—I can walk, I can type, I can see the birds, I can hear Beethoven. I came away from that exercise simply not feeling like a sick person. In fact, I realized that the more I believed the thought, "I am sick," the sicker I felt.

By offering us a systematic method for examining thoughts that are a source of suffering, Byron Katie's inquiry takes us to the Buddha's second noble truth: the origin of suffering is desire. Behind every stressful thought is the desire for things to be other than they are. I wanted friends to visit. I wanted to go to Spirit Rock to see Katie. I didn't want to be sick. These "four questions and a turn-around" give us a tool for making peace with our life as it is.

13

Healing the Mind by Living
in the Present Moment

When we settle into the present moment,
we can see beauties and wonders right before our eyes—
a newborn baby, the sun rising in the sky.
—THICH NHAT HANH

WHEN PEOPLE first realize that they have a chronic condition that's going to severely restrict their activities, they'll try just about anything to get their old lives back: prescription drugs, homeopathic medicine, esoteric mind-therapy techniques, nutritional supplements, even oxygen chambers. When the Parisian Flu settled into a chronic illness, I scoured the Internet looking for possible treatments. (I have a big carton that I refer to as "the box of rejected supplements.")

My online wanderings revealed that many people, regardless of their religious affiliation, found that starting a meditation practice was the single most helpful treatment they'd tried. So, Buddhist or not, many people turn *to* meditation when they become chronically ill. This devoted Buddhist, however, turned away from it.

When I got sick, I had a ten-year established sitting meditation practice. I meditated twice a day for 45 minutes each time, following the traditional instruction to be "mindful of in- and out-breathing"—sometimes called "following the breath." When my mind wandered from the breath (perhaps to thoughts about all I had to accomplish the next day), I'd gently bring my attention back to following the breath again. This is one of the basic instructions given by mindfulness meditation teachers. The purpose of the instruction is to keep returning our attention to our experience of the present moment.

I was so disciplined, and stubborn, regarding this practice that it had become a part of our family lore to recall—and to tease me about—how on our daughter's wedding day in 1996, I still managed to get in my two formal sittings. What made this remarkable was that, although Mara and Brad lived in Washington, D.C., the wedding was in Davis where Mara grew up. She and Brad arrived in Davis two days before the festivities. I have never been a party giver. (Tony's and my wedding had twelve people in attendance.) But here I was, non-party giver, putting on a wedding for over 150 people. Needless to say, I was overwhelmed by my responsibilities on the wedding day. But the family knew: whatever else happens on this day, Mom is going to meditate, not once, but twice.

At the Spirit Rock retreat in July 2001, when I awoke on the third day and realized that some form of the Parisian Flu had returned, I raised it at my next teacher interview. I reported that I found it difficult to meditate because I was physically ill. I was told that being sick was the very best time to meditate because it would prepare me for when I was approaching death. I should just follow my breath and note the bodily sensations as they arose. I returned to my room and lay on the bed, trying over and over to meditate, but the sickly bodily sensations were just too unpleasant for me to stay with. I couldn't do it on the retreat and, upon returning home, to the surprise of my family, I discarded that ten-year mindfulness meditation practice that we all thought was set in stone. I felt like a failure whenever I would read online how helpful meditation was to people who were chronically ill. But when I would try, the discomfort of the heart-pounding, crushing fatigue was overwhelming.

It took me seven years to take up mindfulness practice again. I did it by rediscovering the books of Thich Nhat Hanh, whose teachings focus on mindfulness of the present moment, whether in formal meditation or not. Before I say more about Thich Nhat Hanh's teachings, I want to offer two practices that illustrate how "mindfulness of the present moment" can alleviate suffering.

Mindfulness-of-the-Present-Moment Practices

The first practice is a two-part exercise I call "drop it."

Start by consciously taking your mind *out* of the present moment and into the past by remembering something you blame yourself for, you regret, or that simply makes you sad. For me, the sad memory might be of the profession I gave up or of the missed birthday parties for my two granddaughters. Also, there are treatments I regret having tried, and recalling them gives rise to stressful thoughts such as "Am I sicker today because of that potentially toxic antiviral I took for a year with no positive results?" For a caregiver, the memory might be of a trip that had to be cancelled because your loved one was too sick to go.

Now, keep this sad or stressful memory strong in your mind and then . . . *just drop it.*

Maybe you can drop it for only a microsecond, but just drop it and direct your attention to some current sensory input. It could be something you see or hear or smell. It could be the feel of your feet on the ground or the sensation of the breath coming in and going out of your body. Can you feel the relief?

If not, try the exercise again. With practice, you'll find that at the command "drop it," the memory is gone and so is the suffering that accompanied it. With your mind in the present moment, maybe you hear a bird chirping or feel the sensation of a breeze on your body or see a beautiful print on the wall or smell something cooking in the kitchen. As Thich Nhat Hanh says in the epigraph at the head of this chapter, "When we settle into the present moment, we can see beauties and wonders right before our eyes." If you're not having success with this exercise, try it while keeping your eyes closed as you focus on the memory. Then, as you drop it, open your eyes and pay attention to whatever sensory input is there in the present moment.

Now let's move to part two of the exercise. Consciously take your mind out of the present moment by thinking of something in the *future* that you're worried about or that's a source of stress or agitation for you. It could be something personal or it could be thoughts about the future of the world. I have a recurring thought that is a tremendous source of stress—it is the fear that Tony will get ill or have an accident and will need me at his side in the hospital to deal with doctors and to care for him, which I won't be able to do.

I conjure up this fear more often than I'd like to admit. But here's what I do. First, I acknowledge that the fear is there by labeling it: "Ah yes, my old friend, the hospital scare." Then I just drop this conjured thought and direct my attention to a sight, a sound, a smell, or a tactile sensation. Every time I drop this train of thought about the future, I relax into the present moment and the fear and the suffering that accompany the thought lift as if I've shed a heavy weight. I know the thought will be back. But I know what to do when it comes back. (I love Mark Twain's comment on stressful thoughts about the future: "I've lived a long life and seen a lot of hard times . . . most of which never happened.")

In a nutshell, that's the exercise:

Take your mind back in time to a stressful memory, and drop it.

Take your mind forward in time to a stressful thought, and drop it.

You're left in the present moment. Even if that moment is accompanied by bodily pain or discomfort, it will be easier to relax into the discomfort, riding it like a wave, because you won't be making it worse by adding to it the mental suffering that comes with thoughts about the past and the future, such as: "I shouldn't have overdone it yesterday"; "I'm afraid this pain will never go away." I know my mind will wander into that past and future suffering territory again and again, but I also know that I can bring it back to the present moment with a simple "drop it."

I used this practice recently when stressful thoughts about both the past and the future overwhelmed me in a situation which was, in retrospect, quite mundane: It has to do with the time I broke my ankle just after Tony left for a month-long retreat. The ankle healed, but I was left with an uncomfortable swelling and tingling on the ball of my foot and in my toes. My family doctor referred me to a podiatrist. I thought, "This is a treat—a doctor's visit that has nothing to do with my illness!" Tony had a conflicting obligation so, because the podiatrist's office was only a half-mile from the house, I drove myself to the 2:30 appointment.

By 3:00, I was on the examining room chair, my mind spinning with a list of grievances about the past thirty minutes and in irritation about the future. First, the person who scheduled the appointment over the phone had given me faulty directions to the office so I drove in circles for ten minutes, worrying that I'd be late. Second, once I found the place, I had to sit in the waiting room for more than twenty minutes. Third, the person who showed me to the examining room said the doctor was currently seeing a patient and had one other person ahead of me. Fourth, the special podiatry examining room chair appeared to be designed for my discomfort!

Angry about the past thirty minutes, irritated about the future (*Just how long would it be until the doctor came in?*), I closed my eyes, took a deep breath and silently said, "Drop it." In the space created by those two words, the thought arose that I knew nothing about the room in which I sat. The idea came to me to open my eyes and look carefully at the room. What color were the walls? Did the room have the same kind of false ceiling that I came to know so well as I lay on the couch in my law school office? What tools of the podiatrist's trade might be lying around for me to visually inspect from the chair? Was there a picture on the wall? Was there a window in the room?

I opened my eyes and began to mindfully explore this space. As I was doing this, my anger and irritation vanished. In fact, the exploration was so thoroughly absorbing that when the doctor came in to see me, it felt too soon because I hadn't yet finished examining the details of the collage on the wall!

This practice is a variation of an instruction we're given when learning formal meditation practice. When our mind wanders away from mindfulness of in- and out-breathing, away from the awareness of the physical sensation of the breath going in and out of the body, we are told to gently bring our attention back to awareness of the sensation of the breath. Those mental wanderings take us to thoughts about the past or about the future, thoughts that are often a source of suffering. But the actual sensation of the breath is in the present moment. While sitting in meditation, Joseph Goldstein sometimes silently but firmly says "not now" to intrusive thoughts, and then he returns to following his breath. This is similar to the drop-it practice I use outside of formal meditation.

From my daughter Mara, I learned a remarkable practice that is similar to drop-it. It comes from Byron Katie. Mara was listening to a podcast of Oprah Winfrey interviewing Katie in 2008 on the radio show "Oprah and Friends." Katie was sharing a story about her daughter who, years ago, had problems with alcohol and drugs. Her daughter would go out at night in her car and, in the early hours of the morning, Katie would sit and wait for her daughter to return. The later it got, the more stressful Katie's thoughts became. She would imagine her daughter had been raped. She would imagine that her daughter had had a car accident and was dead or was lying injured on the road in agony with no one to help her. Then one early morning, as the thoughts began to arise again, Katie realized that the only thing that was true for sure was this: "Woman in chair, waiting for her beloved daughter."

Mara heard this story and knew it contained a gem, because she started to free her own mind of stressful thoughts and ground herself in the moment by using whatever version of Katie's words applied. In fact, Mara happened to be sharing this story with me because the day before had been a particularly stressful one for her, physically and emotionally (an emergency trip to the dentist for eight-year-old Malia was but one of the highlights). Mara said that as she was lying in bed that night, trying to read, stressful thoughts about the day kept spinning around in her mind. It's as if she were re-living the day over and over. (We've all done this, haven't we?) Then she said to herself: "Woman lying in bed, reading a book." Suddenly, she was, well, just a woman lying in bed, reading a book! She'd brought herself out of the past and into the present moment, just as Katie had brought herself out of thoughts about the future—all the terrible scenarios she was mocking up for her daughter—and into the present moment with "Woman in chair, waiting for her beloved daughter."

The day after Mara shared this with me, I found myself caught up in a repeating round of stressful thoughts about the previous day. I was blaming myself for not having been more disciplined about the amount of time I'd spent socializing with a friend who had come over. Of course, it's not a bad idea to examine the effects of over-socializing on our symptoms, but blaming ourselves and feeling guilty about something that's already happened is not constructive.

"It's your own fault that you feel so sick today," I thought for the dozenth time, at which point I looked up and saw my face in the mirror of the bathroom sink and said, "Woman on stool, brushing her teeth." It was a magical moment. It broke the hold these stressful thoughts had on me. Just to be sure, I repeated (to use Katie's words) the only thing that was true for sure, "Woman on stool, brushing her teeth." And I smiled because being in the present moment is a relief indeed!

The Vietnamese Zen master Thich Nhat Hanh does teach formal meditation practice, but he focuses just as much on staying mindful of the present moment as we engage in activities of everyday life, from brushing our teeth to making the bed to washing the dishes. In *The Miracle of Mindfulness* he offers several exercises in mindfulness. Many of them start with the instruction to "half-smile"—a wonderful practice in itself. Try a half-smile and see how your mind and body immediately relax and how a touch of serenity arises. Here are two of Thich Nhat Hanh's mindfulness exercises, which you can easily apply in your own life:

> *Half-smile while listening to music.* Listen to a piece of music for two or three minutes. Pay attention to the words, music, rhythm, and sentiments. Smile while watching your inhalations and exhalations.
>
> *Mindfulness while making tea.* Prepare a pot of tea. Do each movement slowly, in mindfulness. Do not let one

detail of your movements go by without being mindful of it. Know that your hand lifts the pot by its handle, know that you are pouring the fragrant warm tea into the cup. Follow each step in mindfulness. Breathe gently and more deeply than usual. Take hold of your breath if your mind strays.

I still haven't found a way to resume a "formal" meditation practice even though it was such a major part of my life before I got sick. Nonetheless, I do practice every day with the tools and exercises in this book—including times when I am working to transform my negative self-judgment that sometimes arises from the fact that I no longer "sit" formally. But using drop-it practice, Byron Katie's teaching, and the teachings of Thich Nhat Hanh on mindfulness of the present moment allows mindfulness practice to remain an important part of my life.

I encourage readers to give formal mindfulness meditation a try, if your health and physical condition allow for it. You can find instruction online or in books. Thich Nhat Hanh provides instruction in *The Miracle of Mindfulness*. I also recommend Joseph Goldstein's *The Experience of Insight* and Bhante Gunaratana's *Mindfulness in Plain English*.

If you are not spiritually inclined, look at the work of Jon Kabat-Zinn. He was the pioneer in taking traditional Buddhist mindfulness meditation and turning it into a secular practice. He founded the Center for Mindfulness in Medicine, Health Care, and Society at the University of Massachusetts Medical School and has written several books on using mindfulness meditation to reduce stress and to promote healing in a variety of medical conditions.

If bodily pain or discomfort prove to be obstacles, try guided audio meditations. Because you're listening to a guide's voice, your mind has something to do other than to concentrate exclusively on bodily sensations. Even if the meditation focuses on the body, being guided by a voice makes it easier to relax into sensations without making the discomfort worse by adding stressful thoughts.

I'll close with a prayer that Sylvia Boorstein uses and shares with us in her book *Happiness Is an Inside Job*. While discussing how mindfulness and metta are partners in practice, she says, "I cannot be genuinely mindful—open to my moment-to-moment experience without hesitation or hiding—unless my mind is benevolent . . ."

And she offers this aspirational prayer, which you can say over and over again:

> *May I meet this moment fully.*
> *May I meet it as a friend.*

14

What to Do When (It Seems) You Can't Do Anything

Today, like every other day, we wake up empty
and frightened. Don't open the door to the study
and begin reading. Take down a musical instrument.
Let the beauty we love be what we do.
There are a hundred ways to kneel and kiss the ground.

—RUMI

IN TEACHING US HOW to alleviate or put an end to the suffering in the mind, the Buddha presented the Eightfold Path, which I briefly described earlier. When we were exploring how to handle insensitive or hurtful comments, we discussed cultivating wise speech, and we'll take that up again in the next chapter. But first, we need to look at another practice on the Eightfold Path—wise action—because it has a lot to teach the chronically ill about how to take care of themselves. Simply stated, actions that lead to the cessation of suffering are to be cultivated and actions that enhance or amplify suffering are to be avoided. Wise *inaction* can thus be thought of as simply not engaging in those actions that make our condition worse.

Since becoming sick, I've learned how crucial—yet difficult—it is to practice wise inaction. The challenge is to avoid actions that exacerbate symptoms because worsening symptoms give rise to both physical and mental suffering—sometimes so severe that I break down in sobs of despair, dukkha in abundance, a total meltdown. This used to happen frequently, but now it's a rare occurrence, thankfully. A meltdown is not only hard on Tony, but leaves me feeling even more sick.

Obviously, those of us who are house-bound must let go of activities that take us away from our dwelling place. I am not physically unable to leave the house, but the exacerbation of symptoms that results is seldom worth the journey. Even in the confines of the house and yard, however, it takes tremendous discipline to avoid overexertion. I'm still working to overcome a lifetime of conditioning that led me to believe that making sure my house looked its best was essential to the quality of life of the family. Suddenly and unexpectedly, tasks such as keeping windows washed, surfaces dusted, walkways cleared of leaves, became actions that increased suffering. Every day, I have to muster the willpower to stop myself from doing something that now comes under the category of unwise action, and I don't always succeed. I keep a haiku of Issa's posted nearby. It's about nonharming, but I use it as a reminder to let go.

> Don't worry spiders,
> I keep house
> casually.

The Middle Way

Can we live a good and fulfilling life when our activities are so severely curtailed? Are there actions that can reduce suffering despite the limitations imposed by chronic illness?

I've discovered that wise action lies in finding the middle ground between what we used to be able to do and the alternative of doing nothing, out of fear of exacerbating our symptoms or out of anger over our perceived misfortune. The challenge is to find the "middle way," the balance between too much and too little.

In *A Still Forest Pool*, Ajahn Chah talks about his teaching method. I use his discourse as a guide for determining what is wise action, given my new limitations:

> It's as though I see people walking down a road I know well. To them the way may be unclear. I look up and see someone about to fall into a ditch on the right-hand side of the road, so I call out to him, "Go left, go left!" Similarly, if I see another person about to fall into a ditch on the left, I call out, "Go right, go right!" That is the extent of my teaching. Whatever extreme you get attached to, I say, "Let go of that too." Let go to the left, let go to the right. Come back to the center, and you will arrive at the true Dharma.

The key to wise action for the chronically ill, then, is to avoid extremes. If we veer too far to the one side and act as if we have the stamina and physical abilities we used to have, we risk overexertion that could land us in bed for days. But if we veer too far to the other side of the road (for example, lie in bed in a fetal position as I did for several months early on in my illness), we risk falling into despair. Another extreme. Either one increases our suffering (and that of our caregivers) and so cannot be considered wise action. The challenge is to find that middle ground.

One Thing at a Time

Another guideline for wise action comes from Korean Zen master Seung Sahn. It's a teaching I consider crucial as I try to engage in wise actions from my bed:

"When reading, only read. When eating, only eat. When thinking, only think."

For us, this means "No multitasking!" This is particularly good advice for the chronically ill whose symptoms are exacerbated if there's too much sensory input. It takes a lot of discipline to break our habit of multitasking. Mindfulness practice helps because, unless we consciously pay attention to the present moment, we can find ourselves engaged in multiple tasks without even realizing it.

Help!

Caregivers also find themselves forced into a change in "action" by this new and unexpected life change. Whether they are the spouse, partner, child, or parent of a chronically ill person, activities away from home that were a source of joy may suddenly be severely curtailed because they have to stay home to care for the person in their care. Even at home, their ability to interact and socialize with their loved one may be severely limited by his or her illness.

It's not surprising that caregivers experience moments of despair when they exclaim (out loud or silently), "Help! I just don't know what to do to help make you better." This dilemma takes me back to the theme reflected in the title of this chapter, and so the question becomes "What can caregivers do for their loved one when (it seems) they can't do anything?" Here's what happened in our household.

After I'd been sick for a while, I noticed a change in what Tony was delivering to me in bed each night for dinner. All of a sudden, I was receiving a gourmet meal! Not only did it taste spectacular, but it was aesthetically beautiful to the eye. He'd take great care to include foods of different consistencies and colors. Looking forward to that meal became the highlight of my day. I didn't ask him, but I suspected that he began to do this because he realized he couldn't cure this illness (a dozen doctors couldn't, how could he?), but this was something he *could* do that contributed to my quality of life.

Even if you are helpless to cure your loved one's illness, there are wise actions, kind and generous actions, in which you *can* engage—cooking a meal, giving a massage, reading aloud. I can tell you from experience, these little actions can lift the spirits of a person who is chronically ill—and in so doing, will lift the spirits of the caregiver as well.

15

Zen Helps

Everything
Just as it is,
as it is,
as is.
Flowers in bloom.
Nothing to add.
—ROBERT AITKEN

ALTHOUGH I'M NOT A STUDENT OF ZEN BUDDHISM, I love to read the teachings and commentaries of Zen masters. I'd like to describe for you three ways that Zen has helped me live well with chronic illness—each of which has formed itself into a bit of a practice for me.

First, Zen has a unique ability to shock the mind out of its conventional way of perceiving the world. I can count on Zen to give me a fresh perspective on my own thinking or to take me beyond thinking altogether. Secondly, a core focus of Zen teachings is how little we know for certain. Not only does this encourage me to question my lifelong assumptions, but it also serves as a reminder to stop engaging in that fruitless task of trying to predict what will happen next in my illness (and my life). And, oh, is it liberating to be relieved of the burden of having to know everything! Finally, Zen masters often teach by using poetic forms. As this verse from Soen Nakagawa illustrates, the poetry of Zen inspires us to see the world through new eyes:

> *All beings are flowers*
> *blossoming*
> *in a blossoming universe.*

As a bonus, the Zen way of conveying the Buddha's teachings—whether by shocking the mind, by pointing to how little we know for certain, or by using poetic language—can often set off a good old-fashioned belly laugh for me, the medicinal effects of which are well-documented.

Shocking the Mind

Koans are stories or dialogues from the Zen tradition. They are great mind-shockers because they can't be understood by using conventional thinking skills. The most famous commentator on koans, Mumon (as he is called in Japanese; or in Chinese, Wumen), said that in investigating Zen, we must "cut off the mind road." The mind road is like a groove we've worn into our consciousness. That groove consists of the endless stream of thoughts and stories we repeatedly spin that cloud our ability to experience the world with a fresh mind or, as Shunryu Suzuki famously said, a beginner's mind.

Take this koan:

> A monk asked Ummon, "What is Buddha?"
> Ummon replied, "A dried shit-stick."

Yes, a dried shit-stick. By way of explanation, I'll just say we now use toilet paper instead of sticks for this purpose. There are dozens of commentaries on this one koan. Katsuki Sekida writes this about it:

> The student asks seriously, "What is Buddha?" Perhaps he is imagining the glorious image of the Buddha pervading the whole universe. The answer comes like a blow to smash such an image. This kind of answer is called "breaking the thinking stream of consciousness."

Sekida's reference to the Buddha as a shit-stick smashing our glorious image of him cuts our mind road right off. It takes us out of our conventional way of thinking into a fresh awareness of the way things are. Because a shit-stick brings to mind something permeated with bacteria and viruses, I interpret this koan as meaning that my diseased, aching body is none other than the Buddha and so this body itself can be a vehicle for liberation, for freedom, for awakening. In his commentary on this koan, Robert Aitken invokes a similar image. He recalls a poem he wrote while a prisoner in a Japanese internment camp during World War II:

In fermenting night soil
fat white maggots
steam with Buddhahood.

Reading Aitken's poem, I think of my chronically ill, "fermenting" body, just *steaming* with Buddhahood. With images of shit-sticks and maggots, Zen shocks my mind into seeing that this diseased body can be a vehicle for awakening.

Oh, and this shit-stick koan gives me a good belly laugh!

Robert Aitken's teacher in the Zen path was Koun Yamada, one of the great Zen masters of the twentieth century. His commentary on Zen koans is called *The Gateless Gate*. In his discussion of a koan called "Tozan's Sixty Blows," Yamada tells the story of the ancient Zen master Bokushi, who was known for his severe approach. If a student wasn't ready to receive the teachings, Bokushi would shove him out the door and slam it. One day, Bokushi was pushing his student Unmon out the door and Unmon's leg got caught and broke. Yamada writes:

> "Ouch!" he cried, and in that instant Unmon suddenly attained great enlightenment. Just "Ouch!," nothing else, no subject or object, neither relative nor absolute, just "Ouch!" This was Unmon's great enlightenment.

This story is so inspiring to me! It's a vivid reminder that bringing undivided attention to the physical sensation of pain or to our aching body just might shock the mind into awakening—or at least give us a taste of it. No object. Just life as it is, sickness and all.

Don't-Know Mind

Many Zen koans begin by posing a question:
"If you say there is no self, who is saying that?"
"Does a dog have Buddha nature?"
"What is the self?"
These koans used to frustrate me. Now I treat them as questions without answers. To put a different spin on "No self, no problem," I respond to these koans with "No answer, no problem." I used to react with anxiety and with anger at the world to the question of whether I'll ever get over this mysterious illness. Now, I try to treat it as a koan. "Will I get well?"—four words and a question mark, arising in the mind, with no answer. Treating it as a koan changes

my relationship to this question, which arises periodically whether I want it to or not. It allows me to hold it more lightly and wait for it to pass on through the mind.

"Will this antiviral cure me?" When I'd start a new treatment, attachment to the outcome came right along with popping the new pill. Now I try to treat the question of whether a treatment will cure or even help me as a koan—a question without an answer. The Korean Zen master Seung Sahn called this keeping a "Don't-Know Mind."

Don't-Know Mind is a great survival tool for me. During that period of several sleepless nights, when I began to spin out stressful stories of a life without ever sleeping again, I'd stop and remember Seung Sahn's Don't-Know Mind. As I approached bedtime, I'd silently say, "I don't know if I'll sleep or not, so I won't make an assumption one way or the other." That thought would calm me and soon after beginning to practice with it, I again started to sleep. I got through those difficult days by keeping a Don't-Know Mind and by using the practice described in chapter 10—consciously moving the mind from the unpleasant physical sensation that accompanies a body deprived of sleep to the cultivation of one of the sublime states.

Thich Nhat Hanh comes at this Zen view of life from a different angle. He encourages us to examine each thought or precede each action with the reflection "Am I Sure?" This is a powerful teaching since attachment to views and opinions is such a source of suffering. I discovered the value of Thich Nhat Hanh's teaching many years before becoming sick. It started in the most mundane of settings—in front of a counter at a department store along with several other people, waiting to buy a pair of pants. The clerk looked up and said, "Who's next?" A woman next to me stepped forward. I was about to say politely, "Excuse me, but I was here first," when Thich Nhat Hanh's "Am I Sure?" popped into my mind and so I let the other woman go ahead of me. I was 99% sure I was first, but allowing the other woman to check out before me had the most wonderful effect. It became an act of generosity to her, not just because she'd get out of the store before I would, but because I may have saved her from the embarrassment of mistakenly thinking it was her turn to go to the register. And of course, in the end, was I 100% sure I was there first? No. Just 99% sure.

That mundane setting planted the seed for a practice that is central to my life as a chronically ill person.

"This doctor doesn't want to treat me." Am I sure? Maybe he's just badly overbooked today.

"This friend doesn't care about me anymore." Am I sure? Maybe she's caught up in family or work problems.

"I'll never get better." Am I sure?

"I'm not leading a productive life anymore." Am I sure?

I have used Thich Nhat Hanh's three short words hundreds of times to let go of assumptions and opinions, an act that allows the world to unfold as it will. I find this practice works particularly well in conjunction with Byron Katie's method for investigating the validity of our thoughts.

The Poetry of Zen

Zen teachings tend to be short and to the point. In addition to koans, they often take the form of *gathas*—short verses reminding us of our practice—and haiku. The distinctive style and rhythms of these writing forms are poetic to the ear. They can be insightful, they can be soothing, and they too can make us chuckle.

Gathas help us dwell in the present moment as we engage in tasks of everyday living. In his book of gathas *Present Moment Wonder-*

ful Moment, Thich Nhat Hanh says that gathas are "exercises in both meditation and poetry." Here's his gatha for washing our feet:

> *Peace and joy in each toe—*
> *my own peace and joy.*

and his gatha for throwing out the garbage:

> *In the garbage I see a rose.*
> *In the rose, I see the garbage.*
> *Everything is in transformation*
> *Even permanence is impermanent.*

In my early years of Buddhist practice, when mindfulness of the present moment was new to me, I carried this little gem of a book everywhere.

I also love a book of gathas called *The Dragon Who Never Sleeps* by Robert Aitken. His gathas are indeed exercises in meditation and poetry. Many of them also make me laugh. Poetic mindfulness plus a laugh—great medicine for the chronically ill.

Here's a sampling of Aitken's gathas:

> *When wayward thoughts are persistent*
> *   I vow with all beings*
> *To imagine that even the Buddha*
> *Had silly ideas sometimes.*

> *When traffic is bumper to bumper*
> *   I vow with all beings*
> *To move when the world starts moving*
> *and rest when it pauses again.*

Raking the leaves from my yard
  I vow with all beings
To compost extraneous thoughts ·
And cultivate beans of the Tao.

Haiku is a form of Japanese poetry that follows a set structure. They are a favorite form of expression for Zen masters and Zen students. My favorite haiku master is the eighteenth-century poet Kobayashi Issa. Issa his lost mother at the tender age of two and lost three of his own children when they were infants. And yet the haiku he wrote—especially about little creatures—never fail to make me smile:

Climb Mount Fuji,
O snail,
but slowly, slowly.

> *Mosquito at my ear,*
> *does it think*
> *I'm deaf?*

> > *I'm going out,*
> > *flies, so relax—*
> > *make love.*

I am so moved by how this man, whose life was filled with personal tragedy, could write poems of such careful observation, such creativity, and often of such unbridled joy. I'll close with a haiku from Issa that illustrates all three ways in which "Zen helps":

The world of dew
is the world of dew
And yet, and yet . . .

Issa's poetic use of words enables me to see the world through new eyes—eyes that keep a Don't-Know Mind. "Dew is dew," he appears to assert, but the last line of the haiku tells me that nothing is certain. The fleeting nature of dew is such that almost as soon as we see it, it changes into something else. Finally, the last line of the haiku shocks me out of the mind groove that's worn into my consciousness, that groove of the seemingly fixed identity: sick person. And so I could change Issa's words to:

A sick person
is a sick person
And yet, and yet . . .

Yes, Zen helps.

From Isolation to Solitude

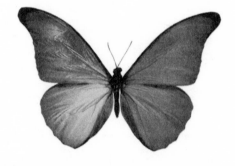

16

Communicating with Care

Take care not to:
talk too much
talk too fast
speak grandly of enlightenment
speak in an obnoxious manner
yell at children
ignore the people to whom you are speaking
speak of things of which you have no knowledge
—RYOKAN, FROM "MY PRECEPTS"

EVEN THOUGH being chronically ill means spending a lot of time alone—which we will delve into soon—we still communicate, just like everyone else. And many of the actions that can cause the greatest suffering or bring about the greatest benefit in our lives are centered on one part of the body: the mouth. Just as the Buddha taught us that we create worlds with our mind, we also create worlds with our speech, so it is important to take great care in how we use it. For the chronically ill, speech—including e-mails, letters, and other written messages—can create support and foster helpfulness or it can increase isolation and alienation.

According to the Buddha, wise speech is endowed with five qualities. It is truthful, spoken with good-will, spoken beneficially, spoken affectionately, and spoken at the right time. These are usually reduced to a formula that contains three considerations:

Speak only when what you have to say is true, kind, and helpful.

It's a tall order to make all our speech true, kind, and helpful, but we can undertake wise speech as a practice by setting the intention to keep those three qualities in mind before we open our mouths. Even Ryokan in the Zen poem in the epigraph that opens this chapter precedes his list of precepts regarding speech with the gentle phrase: "Take care not to . . ." I know that, now and then, I won't speak truthfully and I'll also speak unkindly or in an unhelpful manner. But because I've set the intention to practice wise speech, as opposed to making it a pass/fail commandment, I can forgive myself when I come up short, reflect on my words, and start anew. *Practice* is the operative word. With practice, we can become quite skillful at putting our words through the filter of true, kind, and helpful before we speak out loud—or hit the send button!

I've found that it's often easy to meet two of the criteria, but not all three. For example, it may be true that a friend hasn't been in touch for a month, but would it be helpful to confront the friend about it? Before sending a "Why haven't you been in touch?" email, if we replace the intention to confront with the intention to inquire ("How are you doing?"), the communication might just become kind and helpful. We may discover that the friend hasn't been in touch because he or she is having work or family problems, which gives us the opportunity to respond with compassion and support rather than self-interest.

After becoming chronically ill, I faced an unexpected challenge in practicing wise speech. I assumed that anyone who cared about me would want to know, in detail, everything about the illness and my attempted treatments. For the first five years, after every appointment with a new specialist or after starting a new treatment, I'd write a long, detailed email, which I would then send to Jamal and Mara and a friend or two. In response, I'd typically get a few supportive sentences.

Not only did I assume that those to whom I was closest wanted to know every detail about my illness, but I now believe that on some level I was also trying to make sure they realized just how sick I was. These detailed descriptions passed the Buddha's test of truthfulness, but in sending them out, I wasn't stopping to reflect on whether they were kind and helpful to those receiving them. Yes, I was sick, but everyone's life has its share of suffering—our old friend the first noble truth—and I wasn't speaking wisely when I failed to consider this. If Jamal was in the midst of a painful lower back flare or if Mara was overly busy with the many activities she juggles each day, surely it's neither kind nor helpful to ask them to read and respond in kind to a two-page email that's loaded with medical jargon and a detailed account of my difficulties. I was sick for five years before it dawned on me that I needed to re-evaluate my understanding of wise speech.

When I looked more deeply, I saw that my relationship with family and friends would be richer and more enjoyable for all of us if I didn't always talk about my illness. Included in the notion of wise speech is what the Buddha called noble silence—knowing when *not* to speak. Not only did I stop describing my experience with every new specialist and every new treatment, but I looked for things to talk about with family and friends that would bring interest and joy to our relationship. Now I'm much more likely to ask about their lives instead of talking about my illness.

One time, for example, when I had a cold—"sick upon sick" we call it—I phoned Jamal on a Sunday to say hello. I opened my mouth with the intention to tell him about the cold but caught myself and, instead, asked him what he was up to. We chatted for a half-hour and I never mentioned the cold. I hung up, feeling great about our conversation. It had lifted my spirits and I hope it lifted his.

I don't even share with Tony the details of every treatment—to alleviate symptoms, to help me sleep, or for the long-shot cure. I use notebooks to keep track of how I'm doing, and the entries are crucial because they enable me to see the effects of different drug dosages and the like. But about five years after getting sick, I decided that I didn't want my relationship with Tony to be only about the illness. He's exposed to it every day as it is. (Even when he's out of town, he checks in by phone or email unless he's on a silent retreat.) If I sat him down each day and analyzed my latest notebook entry, he'd listen. But unless I need feedback or advice, sharing with Tony the details of every symptom and response to a treatment would be neither kind nor helpful, even though it would meet the truthfulness test.

Noble silence doesn't spare Tony from listening during my greater moments of need—the occasional 2:00 A.M. sob-soaked outpouring of frustration or the 2:00 P.M. poor me rant as I complain about things I can no longer do. Tony never fails to comfort me when these meltdowns occur. He's the most unselfish person I know.

Chatting

In one source, when asked what constitutes wise speech, the Buddha said to practice abstaining from lying, divisive speech, abusive speech, and idle chatter. The first three are obvious, but the last can be tricky. The Buddha cautioned against idle chatter, not just because it often includes vicious gossip, but because idle chatter— frivolous and meaningless speech—is a distraction from truly important matters such as loving-kindness, mindfulness, and the cultivation of wisdom. In addition, engaging in frivolous talk, even innocent gossip, can give rise to envy and other mental states that are a source of suffering. Having acknowledged the pitfalls of idle chatter, now I must confess: since becoming sick, it's the very type of speech I miss most. Sometimes I long to feel healthy enough to spend a few hours idly chatting away, exchanging trivial anecdotes with family and friends. Chatting can be a way to share a warm exchange and it can lighten the burden of always focusing on serious matters.

My guess is that caregivers also wish they had the luxury to have a chat with people more often. Tony and I live in a small town where he was once an elected official. It's hard for him to go anywhere without encountering someone he knows. I'm aware that he doesn't tell me about all the difficulties he encounters out in the world on his own because he doesn't want to burden me with them, but he did share with me one recurring experience.

When he runs into people in the aisles of the grocery store, they immediately ask, "How is Toni?" He's not going to lie and tell them I'm better, so inevitably he says, "She's about the same." He tells me that this calculated to be short-as-possible response is a conversation killer no matter how lightheartedly he says it. There are lots of grocery aisle topics—idle chatter though they may be— that would be fun for him to engage in: local politics; what our respective children are doing; even the weather! But the fact of my ongoing illness is the elephant in the aisle and it's hard to get around the beast.

No doubt, other caregivers face this dilemma. Tony and I have talked about how he can work around it. He has tried to be the one to initiate the conversation by quickly asking how the other person is doing (he reports mixed success). As soon as he's said, "She's about the same," he's also tried moving to a subject that's topical and has nothing to do with our respective families (he reports better success).

Dividing and Abusing

Idly chatting about how your family is doing or your plans for the next week or the upcoming referendum are usually at worst neutral, but I think a key concern the Buddha had about idle chatter was that it can easily degrade into divisive and abusive speech. Not only can this type of speech harm others, but it can harm the speaker too.

The antonyms for *divisive* and *abusive* are *unifying* and *cordial*, respectively. When we speak cordially to others, with the intent to bring unity to the interaction, we are directing loving-kindness toward them. In this way, wise speech goes hand in hand with our cultivation of the sublime states. We are also being kind to ourselves, since divisive and abusive speech give rise to mental states—envy, anger, resentment—that are sources of mental suffering and—particularly if you are chronically ill—physical suffering.

If you find yourself about to speak divisively or abusively to others, a good antidote is patient endurance. Cultivating patience slows us down, making us more reflective. This enables us to check our speech for the qualities of *true, kind,* and *helpful* before we release it into the world.

Yes, wise speech can be a tall order. Some days, I'm relieved if I can just meet a couple of Ryokan's goals—not speaking obnoxiously and refraining from yelling at children! But then I remember that the Buddha considered wise speech to be an indispensable practice on the path to enlightenment, awakening, liberation, freedom. With that reminder, I redouble my effort to communicate with others only using words that are true, kind, and helpful.

17

The Struggle to Find Community in Isolation

*I never found the companion
that was so companionable as solitude.*

—HENRY DAVID THOREAU

ALL HUMAN BEINGS need the company and support of others. We create our world together. But community can be a tremendous challenge for someone who must spend a lot of time in bed or must suddenly take to bed in spite of plans to be with others. The Dharma places a very high value on community, which is called *sangha*. The word originally referred to the disciples of the Buddha. It then evolved to include Buddhist monks and nuns. Today, *sangha* refers to the entire spiritual community that supports a practitioner on the path to enlightenment or awakening. Many Buddhists say that sangha is the single most important support on their spiritual path. They speak of taking refuge in sangha. Readers of any faith will appreciate the value of sangha—of community—in spiritual life.

Before I got sick, I was active in several Buddhist sanghas. I co-hosted a weekly meditation group with Tony. We used a local meeting hall every Monday night. At least once a month, I would lead the sitting and then give a talk. We also hosted a monthly group at our house in which we discussed Dharma readings that Tony or I chose and distributed each month. The readings were the starting point for a spirited and often humorous two hours of reviewing our lives since we last met. This was sangha at its richest for me. Tony still hosts this group at our house.

We also frequently went to daylong meditation retreats led by teachers, not just from Northern California, but from all around the world. And, twice a year, I attended a ten-day silent meditation retreat, led by many of the teachers I mention in this book. When I got sick, I could no longer participate in these activities, even though the meeting hall is three blocks away and the monthly group is a room away—although if I sit off to the side and mostly listen, I'm sometimes able to join the monthly group for a half-hour. In addition to losing this precious source of spiritual support, I had to adjust to the social isolation that accompanied the illness like night follows day.

Alone and Cut Off

"It's hard to distinguish between the effects of my illness and the effects of isolation," wrote a member of an online support group for people diagnosed with an illness similar to mine. I, too, have days when the isolation feels like the illness itself. People who are house-bound are not just isolated from one-on-one personal contacts. We are often isolated from nature and even from the warm feel of a friendly crowd. Our best bet to see the changing seasons is on the drive to and from a doctor's appointment, but this is often a stress-filled outing. Similarly, our best bet to be in a crowd is in the waiting room at the doctor's office—not the most comfortable or uplifting of settings. I recently read a entry from a woman with chronic fatigue syndrome in which sh said she went to get a blood test a week early just to be around people.

The subject of friendships can be a painful one for the chronically ill. The sudden lack of day-to-day socializing was the hardest adjustment I had to make—even harder than losing my career. It felt as if there were a hole in my heart that was once filled with the sight and sounds of other people. I didn't write the chapters in this book in the order in which they appear, but I *did* write this one last because I was avoiding the difficult task of putting into words the pain of coming to terms with the loss of so many friends. On an Internet site for the chronically ill, one person put it this way: "Friends slipped away slowly." Another said, "All my friends have gone missing."

In 2008, I was looking through the contents of a folder and came across a note I wrote in June 2002. It caught my attention because, since becoming sick, I've read about other people having written similar notes to family and friends after being diagnosed with a chronic illness that is invisible to others—arthritis, lupus, cancer, diabetes, heart disease, fibromyalgia. After writing the note, I copied it, attached two essays from the book *Stricken: Voices from the Hidden Epidemic of Chronic Fatigue Syndrome*, and sent the packet to four close friends:

> *I'm sorry I couldn't join all of you for lunch today as I'd planned. Unless people have known someone in my situation, it must be hard to understand why I can't do everything since I can do some things and since I seem to look fine.*
>
> *So I thought I'd share a couple of essays. One of the*

women is still working, one is not. Both have been diag-
nosed with chronic fatigue syndrome although, as with
me, the doctors don't really know why they continue to
be sick. Their stories are different from mine, but there
are more similarities in our day-to-day experience than
there are differences.

I don't need you to do anything after reading these
essays; I'll just feel better knowing you're aware of
what's going on with me right now. See you soon.

Love,
Toni

All four of these people have dropped out of my life. And so it goes for many of the chronically ill. As I said earlier, Byron Katie's inquiry has helped me cope with the loss of so many friends, but I vividly remember how I felt when I so carefully composed that note in 2002. I was terrified that my friends would "go missing." And that turned out to be the case.

Chronic illness takes its toll on friendships for several reasons. We become undependable as companions, often having to cancel plans at the last minute if it turns out we can't get out of bed on the day of a scheduled commitment. Even if we can visit, it may only be for twenty minutes and that may be too short a time for people to commit to. (Their drive to see us may be longer than the time we're able to socialize.) Some people are uncomfortable being around those who are sick. Some people no longer know what to talk about around us, believing that sharing stories about their activities will make us feel bad. And, living in the world of the sick, we gradually have less and less in common with those with whom we worked and played.

Knowing these reasons doesn't make the isolation any less painful an adjustment as we watch people disappear from our lives one by one, some after dozens of years of friendship. On top of this painful personal experience, we also encounter all the "healthy living" advice that tells us that maintaining an active social life enhances both mental and physical health. And so worry is added to isolation.

As of this writing, I have only one regular non-family visitor and she was someone who was not even a part of my life when I got sick in 2001. I mentioned my friend Dawn earlier—our children went to nursery school together, but when they were teenagers, she and I grew apart and the friendship all but dried up. I hadn't seen her for almost ten years. When she learned I was sick, she began visiting, even if only for twenty minutes—and she's kept it up. When we arrange a visit, we proceed on the assumption that I'll be well enough to see her. Despite her busy life—realtor, wife, mother of three, grandmother of six—if I have to cancel at the last minute, she gracefully accepts the abrupt change in plans. She's simply not bothered by the unpredictability of my day-to-day condition. I know there are other people in town I could invite over for a visit. I don't do it because experience has taught me that most people don't react with the same understanding as Dawn does should I suddenly have to cancel. I've become gun-shy. This is a common dilemma for the chronically ill.

In September 2007, my second granddaughter, Camden, was born. Since then, my daughter-in-law, Bridgett, has been driving up from Berkeley every Thursday afternoon. Unless Tony is here for her to visit as well, Bridgett knows she can't stay very long, but she insists on coming anyway, despite a drive that is longer than the visit. I play with Camden on the bed while Bridgett and I try to fit in a few minutes of adult talk. I am so grateful to her.

These are my most faithful in-person visitors—three ladies spanning three generations!

Far-Away Friends and Nearer-By Family

There is, of course, an alternative to in-person contacts for the chronically ill—the Internet. It can be a rich source for developing friendships. My ability to connect with others in this way is limited because I can't stay on the computer for long without exacerbating my symptoms. That said, I met a woman online with whom I've been communicating daily via email since 2004. Sometimes a message may be only one line: "Too sick to write today."

At first, we wrote about our illnesses, but when we discovered we had more in common than the physical condition of our bodies, the friendship blossomed. We began to share family stories, our own life histories, literature and the arts, a sprinkling of politics, spiritual pursuits, our deepest hopes and fears. The likelihood of JoWynn and I meeting in person is next to none (she lives outside of Baltimore), but the friendship is as rich as they come.

On the other side of the world, I've met Judy who lives in Sydney. We share stories about life on opposite sides of the planet. We followed the 2008 presidential election together, emailing back and forth as the returns came in. It was my Tuesday night and her Wednesday afternoon when, together, we learned that Barack Obama had won. Recently, Judy's husband made a short video of her to show me around her neighborhood. I saw surfers in the ocean and heard the sound of cicadas. The best part for me though was hearing Judy's Aussie accent.

My illness has also changed the nature of my relationships with my family—sometimes even bringing them "nearer-by." Before I got sick, I visited frequently with my grown children. Mara is an hour's plane ride away and Jamal is an hour's drive away. One way I've maintained a close relationship with them despite my new limitations is through Instant Messaging. With IM, I can have live conversations with them! I lie on the bed with my laptop; they use either their computers or their cell phones, and we "talk" back and forth. When Mara and her family visit, sometimes she even IMs me from the living room to share what's going on in the front of the house. In June of 2009, my son-in-law, Brad, graduated from UCLA's Anderson School of Management. As I lay on the bed, thinking about the graduation ceremony I was missing, this message from Mara's cell phone suddenly popped up on my computer screen: "Brad's name was just called and he's walking across the stage!" These interactions with Jamal and Mara are one of the great joys in my life. In fact, because Mara has never liked talking on the phone, I'm in better touch with her now than I was before getting sick.

The Aloneness Spreads

Caregivers may also find themselves socially isolated because their loved one can't accompany them outside the house or apartment. Tony had a first taste of that lifestyle change on our trip to Paris, unaware that it was to become a permanent feature of his life. "I've lost my companion out in the world," he's often said to me. The loss is more profound than just not being able to go to dinner or the movies together. A lot of the sadness comes from those moments of lost intimacy, like the cherished drive home from a party where Tony and I would "debrief" each other about the interactions we'd had—who we enjoyed chatting with, who we hoped to never see again.

Tony and I were blessed to be best friends as we ventured out into the world. Now, in regard to social activities, he's housebound most of the time too. People who would invite us over as a couple rarely invite Tony over by himself. This is a common experience for the partner of a chronically ill person. It's an odd social phenomenon since, when a person is single, couples have no hesitation including him or her in their social activities.

Even at home, caregivers may be isolated from their loved one. Some days, my ability to visit with Tony is severely limited. This puts caregivers at a dual disadvantage. They're not just alone; they're alone with their worries and their frustration at not being able to make their loved one better.

Solitude

The combination of lost friends and the inability to leave the house makes isolation a fact of life for many of us. After getting sick, it took me several years to realize that isolation itself is a neutral state. The dictionary defines it as "The fact of being alone." In the above discussion, I added the words "painful," "sad," "difficult," because that was my experience of isolation in the early years of the illness. If isolation has also been a source of suffering for you, recall the good news that the Buddha delivered in the third noble truth: there are steps we can take to help alleviate suffering in the mind. Relatedly, consider this excerpt from Paul Tillich's *The Eternal Now*:

> Language . . . has created the word "loneliness" to express the pain of being alone. And it has created the word "solitude" to express the glory of being alone.

To examine if this statement could help me change how I react to being alone, I returned to the technique used by Byron Katie that my daughter had shared with me. If you recall, Katie was caught up in a cycle of stressful thoughts about the fate of her daughter who was late coming home. By repeating to herself the one thing she knew for sure—"Woman in chair, waiting for her beloved daughter"—Katie was able to stop the mental suffering and just wait until her daughter returned.

I tried this approach as a way to examine isolation ("the fact of being alone") in the context of Tillich's insight. I realized that the very same fact of isolation—"Woman in chair, alone in the house"; "Man lying on bed, alone in the bedroom"—can be accompanied by the mental state of loneliness or it can be accompanied by the mental state of contented solitude.

My online wanderings have revealed that for some people, isolation results in a debilitating loneliness, which Mother Teresa described as the most terrible poverty. On an NPR program, the spouse of a woman who had been diagnosed with chronic fatigue syndrome described it as "a very lonely disease because of the extreme isolation and the misunderstanding of family and friends due to the ridiculous name."

But for others, isolation makes possible a treasured solitude. Some people value solitude because it allows them to have more control over their lives. A woman in an online support group for the chronically ill, for example, said she loves isolation because it means that no one is making demands on her. Others value solitude because it's an essential part of their spiritual practice. Another woman from the same group said, "Solitude is refreshing to the human spirit and is practiced by all religious denominations to come to know God." Indeed, there is a centuries-old culture of solitude that many people, healthy or sick, find essential to their spiritual well-being despite our culture's emphasis on the necessity of maintaining an active social life.

If you're suffering due to being alone so much, it might help to recognize that being alone in and of itself is not necessarily a negative experience. It's a neutral state—to which we add the desire for things to be other than they are (for example, to have company). When that desire for things to be different goes unfulfilled, we suffer. That's the Buddha's second noble truth: The origin of suffering is desire. Byron Katie's technique can help here too. Bring yourself to the present moment by describing what you're aware of physically: "Woman/Man alone in the house." Then see if without adding the desire for things to be different, you're able to experience a taste of serenity in that aloneness—or maybe just relief that no one is making demands on you! If you can, you'll understand that words like "sad" and "painful" need not necessarily accompany the fact of isolation in your life.

When I got sick in 2001, I had neither this valuable tool offered by Byron Katie nor was I aware of Paul Tillich's statement. I did manage to make the journey from the "poverty" of loneliness to the "glory" of solitude, but it took four years. At first, isolation and loneliness were synonymous for me and I suffered deeply. After the initial six months of acute illness, friends rarely came to see me and Tony was still working full-time. Even after leaving his job, he continued to be busy with work or Dharma-related activities or with trips out of town to see our children and our granddaughter Malia. I spent a lot of time alone—and I cried a lot.

Then one day in 2005, I was listening to an audiobook, *The Dive From Clausen's Pier,* by Ann Packer. At one point, a character said, "Lonely is a funny thing. It's almost like another person. After a while it will keep you company if you let it." And, just like that, in three short sentences, my heart and mind opened to being alone. From that day on, I've been better able to welcome isolation as a friend, and the pain of loneliness has been replaced with the good company of solitude.

Of course, I'm not always successful. Some days, I rejoice in the glory of solitude. Other days I feel so lonely it brings me to tears. Some days, I'm content to let the small town life of Davis unfold without knowing, as I used to, all the details of what's going on socially and politically. Other days, I'm hungry for news from outside the house. Tony is well aware of this latter tendency. Recently, he ran into a woman who did yard work for us many years ago when she was an undergraduate. We knew she'd been through a painful divorce and had been having a difficult time for a few years. To Tony's delight, she told him that she'd met a man and was happily in love. Tony told me that he said to her, "Okay, ask yourself everything that Toni would want to know about him and then tell me, so that I can tell her."

When overcome with loneliness, I use the practices I've described in this book, starting with the first noble truth of dukkha. I recognize that all living beings face suffering. Even those who aren't sick may experience the pain of loneliness. I think of Joko Beck's teaching: This is just my life; there's nothing wrong with it even if I'm lonely at the moment. Then I might move to weather practice, reminding myself that the mental state of loneliness, like everything, is impermanent. It blew in and will blow away, perhaps replaced with the serenity of solitude. Cultivating the sublime states soothes me during these blue periods. Byron Katie's inquiry gives me the tools to examine the validity of stressful thoughts that often accompany the feeling of loneliness, thoughts such as: "Nobody cares about me"; "I'll always be lonely." These Buddhist and Buddhist-inspired practices are always waiting in the wings to help transform that neutral fact of isolation from the despair of loneliness to the serenity of solitude.

The Culture of the Sick

When I told Tony I was writing about sangha, he said that he defines it not just as a person's spiritual community, but as the culture of awakening. I love that view of sangha because it expands it to include resources that are beyond the face-to-face contacts that may have become impossible for the chronically ill to maintain. The culture of awakening includes websites maintained by spiritual communities, talks on CDs, blogs. Just enter "Buddhism" or any religion or other spiritual tradition into Google and you'll be awash in resources that can help substitute for a traditional sangha.

For the chronically ill, another culture can be added to this expanded view of sangha. When I became sick, I felt as if I'd left the culture of awakening and entered the "culture of the sick." (On NPR, essayist Richard Rodriguez talked about entering this "other America" when he was diagnosed with cancer.) When I log on to the Internet to connect with people, I find myself drifting, not to Buddhist websites, but to blogs where people are similarly sick. I've encountered bloggers who range in age from a sixteen-year-old girl with chronic fatigue syndrome who can rarely leave the house, to a mom with multiple sclerosis who is struggling to raise two girls, to a man in his sixties with diabetes who writes a daily blog from his bed.

These people don't use the term *dukkha* (the teenager is a devoted Mormon for instance), but they are writing about suffering. For me, sangha now includes these chronically ill people who have come face to face with the fact of suffering in their lives and who, like me, are struggling to accept it and to cultivate compassion for their own illness and for those they encounter on the Internet. The fact that they don't share Buddhism per se with me doesn't matter—they're part of my sangha.

It's a limited sangha for me because, many days, the computer time I can handle limits me to reading and answering an email or two and checking a few blogs or news sites. But many of the chronically ill aren't as limited. Whatever your illness, it's easy to find support groups and blogs peopled by those facing the same difficulties as you. I know from reading the comments left on the blogs I do follow that these online contacts can be a lifeline. One woman wrote that she was overwhelmed by loneliness until she found blogs written by people who were similarly sick because for the first time since becoming ill, she was able to connect with people who understood her.

The word I used in the title of this chapter, struggle, describes well my experience in adjusting to the loss of my spiritual community, to the loss of so many friends, and lastly, to being alone much of the time. I've largely come through that struggle, but it took time, it took effort, and it took help from a lot of people—the Buddha, his followers, a philosopher, a fiction writer, and ordinary people who have been generous enough to go online and share their experiences as members of the "culture of the sick."

18

And in the End . . .

This very place is the Lotus Land;
This very body, the Buddha.

—HAKUIN

L IVING WELL WITH CHRONIC ILLNESS is a work in progress for me. Some days, I still cry out:

"I can't stand this oppressive, sickly fatigue one more day!"

"I don't care if stressful thoughts exacerbate my physical symptoms!"

"I don't want to hear that laughter coming from the living room!"

"I don't care if this is the Way Things Are: I don't want to be sick!"

When this happens, I "put my head in the lap of the Buddha," as the Dalai Lama suggests, and again take refuge in one of the practices I've shared in this book. The Buddha's teachings and the practices he inspired are always waiting in the wings to see me through. The Buddha continues to inspire me because he never claimed to be anything more than a human being. In fact, the Buddha found pain just as painful as you and I do, as the Buddhist texts take great care to make clear. Consider this passage about an instance when the Buddha was cut by a stone splinter:

> Severe pains assailed him—bodily feelings that were painful, wracking, sharp, piercing, harrowing, disagreeable. But the Buddha endured them, mindful and clearly comprehending, without becoming distressed.

I take this as a reminder that the equanimity and joy we see in the many images of him are within the reach of every one of us. I never stray far from the first noble truth—the fact of dukkha in our lives. I think here too of Joko Beck's teaching that our life is always all right. There's nothing wrong with it even if we have terrible problems. It's just our life.

In the Buddha's time, his monks would carry a bowl with them as they went into the village to collect food from lay supporters. Each day, a monk ate only what was put in the bowl, whether it was filled to the top with scrumptious goodies or contained only a few morsels. Tony uses this as a metaphor for life. We have what is put in our bowl. Tony's and my bowls contain my illness. At times, this has been a great source of suffering for us. But even people whose bowls are usually filled with ambrosia have days when they are only given a few grains of rice. And although Tony's and my bowls contain my illness, our children and grandchildren are in there too, along with other blessings. This is what we've been given.

In October 2009, I was listening to Terry Gross' *Fresh Air* on NPR. She was interviewing country music singer and songwriter Rosanne Cash. Cash had been forced to put her career on hold for several years because she had to have brain surgery for a rare but benign condition. Terry Gross asked her if she ever found herself asking "Why me?"

Cash said "No," that, in fact, she found herself saying "Why *not* me?" since she had health insurance, no 9-to-5 job that she might lose during her long recuperation, and a spouse who was a wonderful caregiver.

Rosanne Cash's words had a profound effect on me. Now, on a day when I start to sink into that "Why me?" mood, I turn it into "Why *not* me?" I, too, have health insurance. I, too, did not suffer financially when I had to stop working, other than having to tighten our budget. I, too, have the best of caregivers. So why *not* me?

I have a Facebook page that I originally created so I could play Scrabble with my family. But gradually I've accumulated "Facebook friends," some of whom I don't know personally because they're friends of my children. In 2009, Davis was the starting point for Lance Armstrong's first race in the U.S. after coming out of retirement. In a town as small as ours, this was a major community event. Our local newspaper expected big crowds to gather downtown for the noontime start of the race despite it being a rainy day. People would be there whom I haven't seen for years. Feeling frustrated, cranky, and lonely because I couldn't be part of this social gathering, but also not wanting to whine online, I posted on my Facebook page "Lying in bed, watching the rain." My daughter's friend, Stephanie, who doesn't think of me as sick because we've never met, added this lovely comment to my post: "That sounds *perfect*!"

I momentarily thought, "Yeah, perfect for *you*," but then I smiled, realizing that my life is indeed perfect. There's nothing wrong with it. It's what I've been given. It's just my life.

In sickness or in health, my heartfelt wish is that you be peaceful, have ease of well-being, reach the end of suffering, and be free.

*A Guide to Using the Practices
to Help with Specific Challenges*

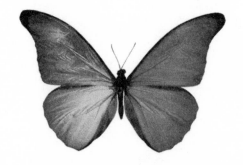

S OME PRACTICES IN THE BOOK may resonate with readers, others may not. I encourage you to try them all and stick with the ones you find helpful.

*Suffering due to the relentlessness of physical symptoms
or from the addition of new medical problems*

▸ *Take solace in the fact that you are not alone*; suffering is present in the lives of all beings. Having been born, we are subject to change, disease, and ultimately, death. It happens differently for each person. This is one of the ways it's happening to you. Recall Joko Beck's teaching: your life is always all right; there's nothing wrong with it, even if you're suffering. It's just your life. The good news from the Buddha is that no matter how much you are suffering physically, there are practices that can help alleviate your mental suffering. (See chapter 3)

▸ *Breathe in the suffering of all those who share the symptoms you're experiencing.* Breathe out whatever kindness, serenity, compassion you have to give. Because you share this particular kind of suffering with them, the thoughts you breathe out will also be directed at yourself. (See chapter 11)

▸ *Repeat the loving-kindness phrases you've settled on,* directing them at yourself, perhaps stroking your body as you do so. (See chapter 7)

▸ *Open your heart to your suffering.* Find words that are specific to the particular difficulty you're experiencing, and repeat them compassionately to yourself: "It's so hard to wake up with a headache every morning"; "It feels overwhelming to have this injury on top of my illness." Recall Thich Nhat Hanh's description of one hand naturally reaching out to the other in pain. Cultivate patient endurance by trying to maintain a calm state of mind while also not giving up on your search for relief from your symptoms. (See chapter 8)

▸ As you experience the unpleasant physical sensations, instead of reacting with aversion, *consciously move your mind toward the sublime state of loving-kindness, compassion, or equanimity*—directing the sublime state at yourself. You can also try moving your mind to *mudita*, taking joy in the joy of those who are in good health. (See chapter 10)

▸ *Try Weather Practice.* Recognize that these physical symptoms are as unpredictable as the weather and could change at any moment. The wind blew the discomfort in and it may blow it out any moment. If a new medical problem develops (like an injury), recall that no forecast of the future could have been certain no matter how many precautions you took. (See chapter 4)

▸ *Try to keep Don't-Know Mind*, reminding yourself that you don't know how long any particular discomfort will last. It won't last indefinitely, and you might even feel better soon. Recall the Zen practice of shocking the mind and how the power of pain could provide such focused attention that the mind is shocked into a moment of awakening. Turn to the poetry of Zen to soothe the body and to feed it the medicine of laughter. (See chapter 15)

▸ *Use Byron Katie's inquiry to question the validity of stressful thoughts* such as "This physical discomfort will never go away" or "I can't stand this symptom one more minute." (See chapter 12)

▸ When a thought persists about the past or future regarding the relentlessness of symptoms ("I caused them because of what I did yesterday...Will they ever subside?"), *acknowledge the thought and then ... just drop it*, bringing awareness to the present moment. Try Byron Katie's practice of stating what you're doing physically *right now*: "Woman lying on bed, resting." This will take you out of your repeating round of stressful thoughts and into the present moment. (See chapter 13)

▸ *Be sure you don't engage in Unwise Action*—actions that could exacerbate symptoms (such as doing too much housework). (See chapter 14)

▸ Recall Munindra-ji's words and recite, "*There is sickness here, but I am not sick.*" Contemplate "Who Am I?" to help shed the fixed identity of "sick person." Try sky-gazing. If you're in bed, try virtual sky-gazing by closing your eyes and shifting your focus from the unpleasant physical symptoms to a more spacious and open experience of body and mind as part of the energy flow of the universe. (See chapter 5)

Blaming yourself for being sick

▸ *Remember that we'd never speak as harshly to others as we do to ourselves,* as Mary Orr discovered. (See chapter 8)

▸ *Breathe in the suffering of all those who blame themselves for being sick.* Breathe out whatever kindness, serenity, compassion you have to give. Because you share this particular kind of suffering with them, the thoughts that you breathe out will also be directed at yourself. (See chapter 11)

▸ *Repeat the loving-kindness phrases you've settled on,* directing them at yourself, perhaps stroking your body as you do so. (See chapter 7)

▸ When you think, "It's my fault for being sick," *acknowledge the thought and then . . . just drop it,* bringing awareness to the present moment. Try Byron Katie's practice of stating what you're doing physically *right now*: "Man sitting in chair, reading a book." This will take you out of your repeating round of stressful thoughts and into the present moment. (See chapter 13)

▸ As you experience the unpleasant mental state of blame, instead of reacting with aversion and self-hatred, *consciously move your mind toward the sublime state of loving-kindness, compassion, or equanimity*—directing the sublime state at yourself. (See chapter 10)

▸ *Recall that anything can happen at any time.* This includes chronic illness. It can strike anyone at any moment despite the best of precautions; it's nobody's fault. Try Weather Practice: Recognize that blame is a mental state as unpredictable as the weather. The wind blew this painful mood in and it may blow it out any moment. (See chapter 4)

- *Use Byron Katie's inquiry to question the validity of stressful thoughts* such as "It's my fault that I got sick" or "It's my fault that I don't get better." (See chapter 12)

- Recall Munindra-ji's words and recite, "*There is sickness here, but I am not sick.*" Contemplate "Who Am I?" to help shed the fixed identity of "sick person." (See chapter 5)

Receiving cursory or dismissive treatment from a doctor or other medical professional

- *Ask yourself, "Am I Sure"?* before deciding that the medical professional didn't want to help you. Maybe the person you saw was overwhelmed with work that day or was experiencing personal problems. If you have a follow-up appointment, try to keep Don't-Know Mind until then. (See chapter 15)

- *Use Byron Katie's inquiry to question the validity of stressful thoughts* such as "This doctor didn't want to treat me" or "This medical person thinks I'm not really sick." (See chapter 12)

If you decide that this doctor or other medical professional did unfairly dismiss you:

- *Recall the sayings "If no one is there to receive it, the letter is sent back" and "Don't stand up in the line of fire,"* from Ajahn Chah. Practically, this means accepting that this is the way he or she relates to you and/or your illness and it's time to move on to another doctor. Then try "Let go a little" practice—taking a baby step toward peace and equanimity each time you repeat Ajahn Chah's phrases. (See chapter 9)

▸ *Breathe in the suffering of all those who have been treated poorly by a doctor or other medical professional.* Breathe out whatever kindness, serenity, compassion you have to give. Because you share this particular kind of suffering with them, the thoughts you breathe out will also be directed at yourself. (See chapter 11)

▸ *Try directing your loving-kindness phrases at the people who treated you poorly* (they come under the category of those who are a source of stress in your life). It can be liberating to wish others well—to befriend them in your thoughts—even though they are being insensitive to you. The odds are high that this medical person has been of help to many others. Be glad for those people. (See chapter 7)

▸ *Open your heart to your suffering.* Find words specific to the particular difficulty you're experiencing and repeat them compassionately to yourself: "It hurts so much to be treated dismissively by a doctor." Cultivate patient endurance by trying to maintain a calm state of mind while also asserting yourself with the aspiration that better treatment will result. (See chapter 8)

▸ As you experience the unpleasant mental sensations of being treated in a dismissive manner by this medical person, instead of reacting with aversion, *consciously move your mind toward the sublime state of loving-kindness, compassion, or equanimity—* directing the sublime state at yourself. (See chapter 10)

- If a painful thought persists about the experience, *acknowledge the thought and then . . . just drop it*, bringing awareness to the present moment. Try Byron Katie's practice of stating what you're doing physically *right now*: "Woman sitting in car after a doctor's appointment." This will take you out of your repeating round of stressful thoughts and into the present moment. (See chapter 13)

Suffering due to the inability to visit with people or participate in family gatherings and other social events

- *Cultivate joy for those who are able to have an active social life and attend special gatherings.* This helps alleviate any envy that might arise. By cultivating joy in the joy of your family or friends who are at a particular event, you may find that you can enjoy the event through those who are there. (See chapter 6)

- *Use Byron Katie's inquiry to question the validity of stressful thoughts* such as "I would have had such a wonderful time at that event" or "I can't stand to be left out of socializing." (See chapter 12)

- *Use Broken-Glass Practice: reflect on how all that arises passes away* and so your ability to socialize and go to events was already broken. These changes will befall everyone at some point in life. This is how it's happened to you. Then remember to look after each moment, cherishing what you still *can* do. (See chapter 4)

- *Open your heart to your suffering.* Find words specific to the particular activity or gathering you're suffering over and repeat them compassionately to yourself: "It's so hard not to be able to join the family for dinner." (See chapter 8)

▶ *Breathe in the suffering of all those who are unable to visit with friends or attend family gatherings.* Breathe out whatever kindness, serenity, compassion you have to give. Because you share this particular kind of suffering with them, the thoughts that you breathe out will also be directed at yourself. (See chapter 11)

▶ As you experience the unpleasant mental sensations of not being able to engage in these activities, instead of reacting with resentment and anger, *consciously move your mind toward the sublime state of loving-kindness, compassion, or equanimity*—directing the sublime state at yourself. You can also move your mind to joy in the joy of those who are able to have an active social life. (See chapter 10)

▶ *Try saying, "This was an activity that I was able to enjoy for X years,"* using the practice inspired by Susan Saint James (whose young son died). (See chapter 9)

▶ *Re-read the discussion about loneliness and solitude.* If it suits you, explore the Internet for alternatives to traditional face-to-face relationships and activities, whether it be finding people who are similarly sick or people with whom you share non-illness-related interests. (See chapter 17)

Feeling ignored by family or friends

▶ *Ask yourself, "Am I Sure?"* before deciding that they are consciously ignoring you. They may be busy at work or sick themselves or concerned that contacting you will exacerbate your symptoms. (See chapter 15)

▸ *Consciously counter this painful mental state by taking immediate action and contacting those who you feel are ignoring you.* It's unlikely they were intentionally ignoring you. (See chapter 8)

▸ *Use Byron Katie's inquiry to question the validity of stressful thoughts* such as "He or she doesn't care about me" or "My family should call more often." (See chapter 12)

▸ *Check your own communication skills.* Have you been complaining too much about your illness or going into too much detail about doctors and treatments? Can you find other subjects to talk about—shared interests and the like? (See chapter 16)

If you decide you really are being ignored:

▸ *Take solace in the fact that you are not alone;* suffering is present in the lives of all beings. Even people who aren't sick struggle in their relationships with family and friends. Recall Joko Beck's teaching: your life is always all right; there's nothing wrong with it, even if you're suffering. It's just your life. The good news from the Buddha is that there are practices that can help alleviate your mental suffering. (See chapter 3)

▸ *Repeat the loving-kindness phrases you've settled on,* directing them at yourself. Then try directing the phrases at these people (they come under the category of those who are a source of stress in your life). It can be liberating to wish others well—to befriend them in your thoughts—even if they are being insensitive to you. (See chapter 7)

- *Open your heart to your suffering.* Find words specific to the particular difficulty at hand and repeat them compassionately to yourself: "It hurts to be ignored by those I love." (See chapter 8)

- *Breathe in the suffering of all those who are being ignored by family or friends.* Breathe out whatever kindness, serenity, compassion you have to give. Because you share this particular kind of suffering with them, the thoughts that you breathe out will also be directed at yourself. (See chapter 11)

- *Try saying, "These were relationships that I was able to enjoy for X years"* or "This was a friendship that lasted for X years," using the practice inspired by Susan Saint James (whose young son died). (See chapter 9)

- If a painful thought persists about lost friendships, *acknowledge the thought and then . . . just drop it,* bringing awareness to the present moment. Try Byron Katie's practice of stating what you're doing physically *right now*: "Woman sitting at table, eating." This will take you out of your repeating round of stressful thoughts and into the present moment. (See chapter 13)

- *Re-read the discussion about loneliness and solitude.* If it suits you, explore the Internet for alternatives to traditional face-to-face relationships, whether it be finding people who are similarly sick or people with whom you share non-illness-related interests. (See chapter 17)

Suffering due to uncertainty about the future

- *Take solace in the fact that you are not alone*; suffering is present in the lives of all beings. This includes suffering over life's uncertainty. Recall Joko Beck's teaching: your life is always all right; there's nothing wrong with it, even if you're suffering. It's just your life. The good news from the Buddha is that there are practices that can help alleviate your mental suffering. (See chapter 3)

- *Try Weather Practice*: Recognize that life is as unpredictable as the weather. Predicting the future is like predicting the weather. Remember Dogen's verse—how the bitterest cold may be setting the stage for something joyful. Indeed, the future could hold a lot of sunshine. (See chapter 4)

- *Try to keep Don't-Know Mind*, reminding yourself that you don't know how long any particular symptom or other concern will last. It won't last indefinitely, and it might change sooner than you think. (See chapter 15)

- If a thought about the uncertainty of the future persists, *acknowledge the thought and then . . . just drop it*, bringing awareness to the present moment. Try Byron Katie's practice of stating what you're doing physically *right now*: "Man lying on bed, resting." This will take you out of your repeating round of stressful thoughts and into the present moment. (See chapter 13)

- *Use Byron Katie's inquiry to question the validity of stressful thoughts* such as "I'll never get better" or "The future only holds pain for me." (See chapter 12)

▸ As you experience the unpleasant mental sensation of uncertainty about the future, instead of reacting with worry and fear, *consciously move your mind toward the sublime state of loving-kindness, compassion, or equanimity*—directing the sublime state at yourself. (See chapter 10)

Coping with the disappointment of failed treatments

▸ *Open your heart to your suffering.* Find words specific to the particular difficulty you're experiencing and repeat them compassionately to yourself: "It's so hard to be disappointed yet again." Cultivate patient endurance by trying to maintain a calm state of mind while also not giving up on the possibility that future treatments may help. If you're blaming yourself for the failure, remember that we'd never speak as harshly to others as we do to ourselves, as Mary Orr discovered. (See chapter 8)

▸ *Repeat the loving-kindness phrases you've settled on,* directing them at yourself to soothe you in your disappointment. (See chapter 7)

▸ *Breathe in the suffering of all those who have been disappointed by the results of a treatment.* Breathe out whatever kindness, serenity, compassion you have to give. Because you share this particular kind of suffering with them, the thoughts you breathe out will also be directed at yourself. (See chapter 11)

▸ When a thought about a past treatment persists ("I never should have tried it . . . I should have listened to my friend who warned me the treatment would fail"), *acknowledge the thought and then . . . just drop it,* bringing awareness to the present moment.

Try Byron Katie's practice of stating what you're doing physically *right now*: "Woman lying on bed, reading a book." This will take you out of your repeating round of stressful thoughts and into the present moment. (See chapter 13)

▸ *Try looking at your disappointment the way Ajahn Jumnian would: If the treatment worked, that would have been fine. It didn't so that's fine too; it isn't what your body needed.* Try Ajahn Chah's "Let go a little" practice—taking a baby step toward peace and equanimity each time you repeat his phrases. (See chapter 9)

Handling caregiver burnout

▸ *Take solace in the fact that you are not alone*; suffering is present in the lives of all beings. Recall Joko Beck's teaching: your life is always all right; there's nothing wrong with it, even if you're suffering due to your extra responsibilities. It's just your life. The good news from the Buddha is that there are practices that can help alleviate your mental suffering. (See chapter 3)

▸ *Breathe in the exhaustion and frustration of all those who are shouldering the responsibility of caring for a chronically ill person.* Breathe out whatever kindness, serenity, compassion you have to give. Because you share this particular kind of suffering with them, the thoughts you breathe out will also be directed at yourself. (See chapter 11)

▸ *Try to keep Don't-Know Mind,* reminding yourself that you don't know how long your loved one will need this extra attention. He or she might even feel better soon. Turn to the poetry of Zen to soothe your exhaustion and to feed it the medicine of laughter. (See chapter 15)

▸ *Open your heart to your suffering.* If you're feeling that family and friends could be helping more but aren't, take compassionate action toward yourself by immediately making contact with them. Often people are just waiting to be asked to help but won't make that first contact. Cultivate patient endurance by trying to maintain a calm state of mind while also not giving up on the possibility that future treatments may help. If you're blaming yourself for not being a good enough caregiver, remember that we'd never speak as harshly to others as we do to ourselves, as Mary Orr discovered. (See chapter 8)

▸ *Think of activities you could engage in that might be fun and relaxing for you or for you and your loved-one together.* (See chapter 14)

▸ *Look for ways to talk to others about subjects of interest that aren't related to your loved-one's illness.* (See chapter 16)

▸ If it suits you, *explore the Internet to see if you can find support groups or blogs written by people who are also in the role of caregiver.* (See chapter 17)

▸ *Contemplate "Who Am I?"* to help shed the fixed identity of "caregiver." (See chapter 5)

With Gratitude

Mara Tyler—my daughter. Mara is the first person who told me I should write a book. Without her encouragement, I doubt it would have happened. She's the person I turn to when I'm struggling with being sick and Tony isn't available or I don't want to burden him. She listens and responds compassionately. I feel heard and that allows me to pick myself up and return to the practices in this book. I'm so blessed that she's my daughter.

Jamal Bernhard—my son. Jamal takes me as I am and that relieves me of a tremendous burden. If I can visit in-person, that's fine. If I can't, that's fine. If I can talk on the phone, fine. If not, we'll talk when I'm able. I can call him up, tell him I'm good for five minutes and ask him to give me the scoop on the Super Bowl. He clocks in precisely at five minutes, we exchange Love You's, and I hang up knowing exactly what to look for in the game. Jamal doesn't treat me like I'm sick and that makes our relationship truly special.

Bridgett Lawhorn Bernhard—my daughter-in-law. I wrote about her weekly trip to Davis so I can see my granddaughter, Camden Bodhi, who was born after I'd been sick for six years. Bridgett comes even when Tony is out of town and I may be too sick to visit for long. On those days, after she's left, I'll discover that the garbage has been taken out or that the dishes have been done. I see more of her now than I did before I got sick. She has become a close and treasured friend.

Brad Tyler—my son-in-law. I rarely get to see Brad because his work keeps him in Los Angeles and my illness keeps me in Davis. His wife may be an adult, but she's still my daughter and I think about her well-being all the time. Brad is such a loving and devoted husband and such a hard-working provider for his family that his presence in my life gives me one less thing to worry about, and this brings me joy.

Malia—Mara and Brad's daughter. Malia was born five months before I got sick. She lights up my life even though I'm rarely able to see her. All I need to hear is "Hi Nana" over the phone once in a while, and my heart is full. I'm especially grateful to her for the good company she's been for Tony, her Papa. They adore each other and when he's with her, his spirits are always lifted, giving him respite from his difficult role as caregiver for me.

Camden—Jamal and Bridgett's daughter. Oh, that special moment when I come out of the bedroom and she smiles at me. Cam is new life, fresh life. She makes me glad to be alive.

Sylvia Boorstein—a founding teacher of Spirit Rock. Sylvia helped me learn to treat this illness with kindness and compassion. She also gave me invaluable support and help in moving the book from the manuscript stage to the publishing stage. My deepest gratitude to her is for the good friend she's been to Tony since I got sick. Those of you who have had the good fortune to know

Sylvia will understand what I mean when I say that being in her "presence" (whether in person, by phone, or by email) is like being sprinkled with angel dust.

Dawn Daro—my faithful friend. Our children grew up together, but then Dawn and I grew apart. When she learned I was sick, she called me and began to visit once a week, even if only for twenty minutes. Her steady presence in my life enriches it tremendously.

Richard Farrell—an undergrad with Tony and me at UC Riverside in the 1960s. After being out of touch with each other for over a decade, he recently moved back to Davis. It has rekindled the deepest of friendships. We can count on him. I hope he knows that he can count on us.

Freddie Oakley, Jessica Sevrin, Nhi Nguyen, Jim Schaaf, Joan De Paoli, and others in Davis who, in my absence, keep Tony company out in the world. They meet him for a chat over coffee. They go out to lunch or dinner with him. And they are the people I know I can call on in an emergency when Tony is out of town.

Dr. Paul Riggle—my primary care physician who (as I like to tease him) drew the short straw when my doctor unexpectedly left while Tony and I were on that trip to Paris and I was randomly reassigned to him. Let me count the ways he is a gem: he listens, he never rushes me, he's open to new treatments, he's up to the challenge of having a patient he cannot "fix," he's compassionate. All this while having a huge patient load and a family of his own. He is the gold standard for doctors. He has never let me down. Never.

Deans Rex Perschbacher and Kevin Johnson—the dean and the associate dean of UC Davis School of Law at the time I got sick.

(Rex has since returned to teaching and Kevin is now the dean.) Until my body just plain gave out, Rex and Kevin did everything they could to accommodate my illness, from allowing me to choose the best time of day to teach to replacing some classroom duties with administrative ones that I could perform from the bed. I'm grateful for their efforts.

Josh Bartok—my editor at Wisdom Publications. Josh's initial enthusiasm for the book and his encouragement all along the way carried me on days I felt too sick to complete the project. My only regret is that we have not met in person for surely someone so capable, perceptive, patient, and reassuring would be a pleasure to spend the day with.

Wisdom Publications—a special thank you to everyone for their wholehearted commitment to the book—especially Joe Evans and Ernie Fernandez who worked so hard on promoting it. I'm also grateful to Phil Pascuzzo for his exquisite cover design and to free-lance editor Barry Boyce, who so beautifully polished the manuscript in its final stages.

All my Dharma teachers—from those I've met in person to those I've studied under through their books. Thank you for the gift of the Dharma.

Bibliography

Aitken, Robert. *The Dragon Who Never Sleeps*
———. *The Gateless Barrier*
Beck, Joko. *Everyday Zen*
Boorstein, Sylvia. *Happiness Is an Inside Job*
Buddhadasa, Bhikkhu. *Heartwood of the Bodhi Tree*
Carrithers, Michael. *Buddha: A Very Short Introduction*
Chah, Ajahn. *Food for the Heart*
———. *A Still Forest Pool*
Chödrön, Pema. *The Wisdom of No Escape*
Collins, Steven. *Selfless Persons*
Dass, Ram. *Miracle of Love: Stories About Neem Karoli Baba*
———. *The Only Dance There Is*
Goldstein, Joseph. *The Experience of Insight*
Goldstein, Joseph and Jack Kornfield. *Seeking the Heart
of Wisdom*
Gunaratana, Bhante Henepola. *Mindfulness in Plain English*
Hart, William. *The Art of Living: Vipassana Meditation as
taught by S.N. Goenka*
Hass, Robert, editor. *The Essential Haiku: Versions of Basho,
Buson, and Issa*

Kabat-Zinn, Jon. *Wherever You Go There You Are*

Katie, Byron. *Loving What Is*

Khema, Ayya. *Being Nobody, Going Nowhere*

———. *When the Iron Eagle Flies*

Kornfield, Jack. *Living Dharma*

Levine, Stephen. *A Year to Live*

Macy, Joanna. *World as Lover, World as Self*

Nhat Hanh, Thich. *The Diamond that Cuts Through Illusion*

———. *The Miracle of Mindfulness*

———. *Old Path White Clouds*

———. *Present Moment Wonderful Moment*

Nyanaponika, Thera. *Great Disciples of the Buddha*

Nyoshul Khenpo, Rinpoche. *Natural Great Perfection*

Rahula, Walpola. *What the Buddha Taught*

Richmond, Lewis. *Healing Lazarus*

Rumi, Maulana. *The Essential Rumi*, Coleman Barks with
    John Moyle, translators

Ryokan. *Dewdrops on a Lotus Leaf*, John Stevens, translator

Salzberg, Sharon. *Lovingkindness*

Sekida, Katsuki. *Two Zen Classics*

Seung, Sahn. *Only Don't Know*

Sogyal Rinpoche. *The Tibetan Book of Living and Dying*

Sumedho, Ajahn. *The Mind and the Way*

Suzuki, Shunryu. *Zen Mind, Beginner's Mind*

Tarrant, John. *The Light Inside the Dark*

Yamada, Koun. *The Gateless Gate*

Index

Opening heart to suffering, 58, 69–
70, 166, 170, 171–72, 174, 176,
178
Opera, 49, 82
Orr, Mary, 59, 61, 168, 176, 178

P
Palin, Sarah, 54–55
Past, regrets about, 113–14, 167
Paticca-samuppada ("wheel of suffering"), 90–95
Patient endurance (*khanti*), 64–69,
144, 166, 170, 176, 178
Poetry of Zen Buddhism, 132–35,
167, 177–78
Practices, xiv–xv, 35, 46, 47–48,
165–78
accepting things as they are, 23,
80–82, 84–85, 172, 174, 177
acting on generosity immediately,
61–62
"am I sure?", 131–32, 169, 172–73
appreciating that one had enjoyed
activities for years, 84–85, 172,
174
blaming oneself for one's illness,
not, 59–60, 68, 168–69, 176
breathing in suffering/breathing out
kindness, etc. (*tonglen*), 97–101,
165, 168, 170, 172, 174, 176, 177
"broken-glass", 33–35, 171
caregiver burnout, handling,
177–78
disappointment of failed treatments,
coping with, 176–77
dismissive treatment from medical
professional, handling, 169–71
"don't-know mind", 130–32, 135,
166–67, 169, 175, 177–78

"drop it", 113–16, 119, 167, 168,
171, 175, 176–77
equanimity, 80–85
family and friends, handling problems with, 171–74
"half-smile", 118
"inquiry," Byron Katie's, 104–10,
132, 148, 155, 167, 169, 171,
173, 175
"let go a little", 82–84, 169–70,
177
loneliness, coping with, 152–55
loving-kindness phrases, 51–54,
165–66, 168, 173, 176
mindfulness of the present moment,
113–20
only thing true for sure in present
moment, 116–18, 119, 152–53,
154, 167, 168, 171, 174, 175,
176–77
opening heart to suffering, 58,
69–70, 166, 170, 171–72, 174,
176, 178
opposite action in response to negative impulse, 61–64, 173
patient endurance, 64–69, 144, 166,
170, 176, 178
physical symptoms or medical
problems, coping with, 165–67
"putting head in lap of the Buddha", 159
"sky-gazing", 42, 167
stroking arm with hand of other
arm, 59, 94, 165–66, 168
sublime states, directing at one's
self, 92–95, 166, 168, 170, 172,
176
suffering present in lives of all
beings, 22–23, 165, 173, 175, 177

About the Author

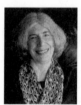 TONI BERNHARD fell ill on a trip to Paris in 2001 with what doctors initially diagnosed as an acute viral infection. She has not recovered.

In 1982, she'd received a J.D. from the School of Law at the University of California, Davis, and immediately joined the faculty where she stayed until chronic illness forced her to retire. During her twenty-two years on the faculty, she served for six years as Dean of Students.

In 1992, she began to study and practice Buddhism. Before becoming ill, she attended many meditation retreats and led a meditation group in Davis with her husband.

She lives in Davis with her husband, Tony, and their hound dog, Rusty.

Toni can be found online at www.tonibernhard.com.

About Wisdom

WISDOM PUBLICATIONS is the leading publisher of contemporary and classic Buddhist books and practical works on mindfulness. Publishing books from all major Buddhist traditions, Wisdom is a nonprofit charitable organization dedicated to cultivating Buddhist voices the world over, advancing critical scholarship, and preserving and sharing Buddhist literary culture.

To learn more about us or to explore our other books, please visit our website at www.wisdompubs.org. You can subscribe to our eNewsletter, request a print catalog, and find out how you can help support Wisdom's mission either online or by writing to:

Wisdom Publications
199 Elm Street
Somerville, Massachusetts 02144 USA

You can also contact us at 617-776-7416 or info@wisdompubs.org.

Wisdom is a 501(c)(3) organization, and donations in support of our mission are tax deductible.

Wisdom Publications is affiliated with the Foundation for the Preservation of the Mahayana Tradition (FPMT)